ANIYS HENDRY

Dr. Sebi's Alkaline and Anti-Inflammatory Diet for Beginners

Discover the Secrets of Dr. Sebi's Alkaline-Anti-Inflammatory Diet. The Easy, Fast and Stress-Free Plant Based Diet.

First edition

ISBN: 978-1-914112-47-8

This book was professionally typeset on Reedsy.
Find out more at reedsy.com

Contents

1

Introduction

We need to change the diet that has been spread by Western globalization. The target groups are hybrids, genetically modified meat, dairy products, processed foods, and plant foods. The use of alkaline plant foods is encouraged. We should analyze agricultural yields in Africa or other parts of the world with similar or similar environmental conditions to Central and South America, the Caribbean, and India.

To support all organs and functions' healing and homeostasis, we need to return to a diet that focuses on whole, non-hybrid plant foods. It is the basis of health and medicine. To accelerate the healing or reversal of complex diseases, we need to reuse natural, essential, and non-hybrid plant ingredients. Dr. Sebi herbal medicine plays a critical role in restoring the notion that non-hybrid plant foods contain chemical compounds for the body and promote healing. The African mineral balance healing method is based on the assumption that the root of the disease is any food that increases the acidity of the body and causes the production of excess mucus in the body. In essence, foods that contain acids and toxins invade the body, creating long-term inflammatory reactions and causing chronic inflammation. Sleep inflammation is a natural, health-promoting process to fight infection and repair physical damage to the body. If acute inflammation is not removed, the process attacks healthy cells in different parts of the body and leads to various diseases. It affects the mucous membranes of the protective organs and promotes excessive mucus production, which affects the organs' health. Therefore, we must begin to eliminate these foods from our diet, including meat, dairy products, processed foods, and unnatural hybrid foods.

Dr. Sebi's diet is not about losing weight, although you can lose weight by following it. Western cuisine is not prepared for your meal; it has fried foods rich in salt, sugar, fats, and calories. In its place, a vegetarian diet is recommended. Herbivores have a higher risk of obesity and heart disease compared to Western diets. Many foods in this diet include calories, fruits, nuts, avocados, and fats. Even though you eat many processed foods, you don't need too many calories and weight.

Consequently, low-calorie foods are not sustainable. Most people who follow this diet are overweight and return to normal health. Because these foods do not define weight and size, it is difficult to know if they contain enough unhealthy calories.

If you want to stop the disease, eliminate the mucus. Also, order some "electric" foods and agree to eat these ingredients to stay alive. He paid particular attention to pH measurements and mentioned that alkaline foods contain more bright energy. There are several gaps in the alkali and viscous theory. In the end, I learned in school that the immune system produces mucus to fight disease and that cardiovascular digestion and respiration depend on our acid production. But I am not a scientist or a doctor. I write a diet that makes black people feel better, and I hope they feel better even when I don't have a chronic illness or painful surgery. I usually punish myself because I am no longer weak.

All plants contain nutrients and phytochemicals and have certain health benefits. Medicinal plants and edible plants or herbs differ from vegetarian foods due to their higher nutrient content. They produce a very bitter or very aromatic or spicy taste. Medicinal plants, such as the Cardo Santo or the "big man," come mainly from flowers, roots and are generally bitter and more effective at fighting disease than food ingredients. Diet herbs such as rosemary and thyme are derived primarily from the leaves of the plants leave, and a small number of these plants are very fragrant or spicy. Due to their higher nutrient and nutrient content, these ingredients are sometimes used in higher doses and act as medicinal plants in traditional medicine.

Plants support the health of the body in two ways. They provide various minerals, vitamins, carbohydrates, fats, and proteins in conditions that naturally support the body's healthy relationship. The organism can replace nutrients lost through metabolic processes that support organ function. Second, the body can use plant esthetics, specific chemical compounds that various plants use to protect themselves against disease. In Africa and similar environments, there are many naturally produced plants. Health is achieved by stopping the intake of other foods while the body is saturated with natural plants. These plants have a chemical affinity for the body and promote the spread of disease. The healthy African genome's expression Science has identified that some people have a genetic tendency to put them at risk from certain conditions. Still, science also claims that environmental factors, such as the food you eat, play a more significant role in determining genes.

2

Chapter 1: Herb List

No eating plan would be complete without a few herbs to make your food more enjoyable by making it taste better. You might even discover that you like food you used to hate if it has the right kinds of seasonings.

Herb List

Burdock – This is a root plant that has been used for centuries in traditional medicine to treat indigestion and fluid retention. Burdock is rich in antioxidants that can prevent some forms of cancer and remove toxins from your body. The root has antibacterial and anti-inflammatory properties, so it is often mashed and mixed with water to treat skin irritations. You can roast fresh burdock root, sprinkle the dried powder on soups and veggies, or steep chunks of the root in boiled water to make tea.

Chamomile – This herb has also been used for centuries in traditional medicine, especially when drinking tea. The antioxidants can help prevent many chronic diseases. It has compounds that will ease your digestive issues and help you fall asleep quickly and sleep deeply. Chamomile tea is an excellent alternative to other teas because it is free of caffeine.

Elderberry – This is another of the medicinal herbs with centuries of use worldwide, especially to treat skin irritations and infections. It can also be used to defend you from viruses and the symptoms of the common cold. Elderberries are high in fiber and vitamin C. The antioxidant content makes them ideal for preventing heart disease and easing inflammation.

Fennel – Fennel bulbs and seeds can be used in cooking and for medicinal purposes. Fennel is low-calorie and rich in minerals, vitamins, and antioxidants, especially vitamin C. The polyphenols in fennel work to reduce the inflammation in your body, and fennel seeds can help to suppress your appetite. Certain compounds in fennel act as antibacterial agents. Roast fennel bulbs with other root veggies or chop them raw and add them to salads. Stir the seeds into soups and sauces.

Ginger – This little root is one of the most delicious and healthiest spices in the world. For centuries, ginger root has been used medicinally to fight off viruses like the common cold and the flu, ease digestive issues, and reduce nausea. Regular consumption of ginger will reduce the muscle soreness and pain associated with exercise, and it can also relieve the symptoms of arthritis. Active compounds in ginger can inhibit the brain's inflammatory responses, leading to loss of function and degenerative diseases.

Raspberry – These berries are low in calories and high in antioxidants, minerals, vitamins, and fiber. Red raspberries are both sweet and tart. The antioxidants will help prevent the development of many chronic diseases. The anti-inflammatory compounds may reduce the symptoms of arthritis, and they may help to decrease your appetite. Eat raspberries by themselves, add them to cereals and salads, or toss them into a smoothie.

Tila – This is also known as linden, and tea has been used as a powerful sedative for centuries. The antioxidants help to fight inflammation and mild chronic pain. Tila may also help promote the excretion of excess fluids to relieve bloating. It can ease upsets of the digestive tract.

Herbal Teas

Burdock Tea – Select some fresh chunks of burdock root. They need to be somewhat firm and not too soft. The color can range from a light color like parchment paper to a dark brown that looks like tree bark. Only buy the root you can use immediately for tea because they do not keep very well. Any leftover root should be put into a soup. You could rinse it well if you chose a younger root, but an older root will need the outer skin scraped off. If you can't source fresh root, you can use one tablespoon of dried root that has been aged for at least one year. If you are using fresh root, then you will need two tablespoons of the root coarsely chopped. Boil the root with three cups of filtered water, and then let it simmer for thirty minutes. Move the pot from the heat and allow the tea to steep for another thirty minutes. Drink the tea to detox your body

Chamomile Tea – This is an herbal infusion made from the dried flowers of the chamomile plant steeped in water. Only Roman Chamomile and German Chamomile are used to make tea. This tea is naturally devoid of caffeine and is often used as a sleep aid. Gather four tablespoons of fresh chamomile flowers, one small sprig of fresh mint, and eight ounces (one cup) of boiling water. Chamomile flowers should ideally be used the same day they are harvested to get the best flavor and medicinal benefits. You will want a tea ball, tea infuser, or a cheesecloth pouch to put the chamomile flowers and mint sprig in. Boil the water and then add in the flowers and mint. Allow the tea at least five minutes to steep. If needed, you can put the mint sprig and the chamomile flowers directly into the water while you boil and steep the tea, and then strain the tea well before drinking. Drink this tea to help you sleep.

Elderberry Tea – This is a delicious tea with the power to boost your immune system. Gather two cups of filtered water, one teaspoon of honey, one-half teaspoon of turmeric powder, one-half teaspoon of cinnamon, and two tablespoons of dried elderberries. Place the elderberries into a small saucepan with filtered water and blend in the cinnamon and turmeric. Please bring this to boiling and then let it simmer for fifteen minutes. The simmering will help to bring out the healing properties of the elderberries. Strain tea water into a cup and blend in the honey as you desire. If you prefer this tea to be served cold, refrigerate it after straining or pour it over ice cubes. Drink elderberry tea when you feel a cold or flu coming on.

Fennel Tea – This is an excellent tea to drink when you have a digestive upset. Gather two teaspoons of fennel seeds, one cup of water, one teaspoon of dried lemon verbena, and one teaspoon of ginger that has been freshly grated. Crush the fennel seeds to release their healing compounds. Peel the chunk of ginger before you grate it. Add all of the ingredients into the water in a small saucepan and boil, and then let it simmer for ten minutes. Strain the tea and drink it immediately. Drink this tea whenever you need to soothe an upset stomach.

Ginger Tea – This is another tea to boost your immunity. It will also warm you in cold weather without giving you caffeine jitters. Rinse off the ginger root to remove any visible dirt. You don't need to peel the root unless you want to. Slice the ginger root, using about an inch of root for eight ounces of water. Put the water and the ginger root in a saucepan and boil, and then simmer for ten minutes. Strain the hot tea and drop in a slice of lemon and a teaspoon of honey for flavor. Drink ginger tea any time your stomach or digestive system needs a little extra help.

Raspberry Tea – This tea is best served cold to get the best flavor. Use a large pot to boil four quarts of water with one and one-half cups of sugar. Take the pot from the heat and keep stirring until all of the sugar is dissolved. Put in twelve ounces of raspberries, ten regular tea bags, and one-fourth cup of lemon juice. Cover the pot and let all of this steep for ten minutes. Then strain the tea well and serve it over ice or refrigerate the tea until it is cold. Drink this tea to stay well hydrated.

Tila (Linden) Tea – This is one of the most straightforward herbal tea recipes.

7

Add one tablespoon of dried linden flowers in a tea ball or mesh basket to three cups (twenty-four ounces) of boiling water. If you need to put the linden flowers directly in the water, strain them well before drinking them. Cover the container and let the flowers steep for at least fifteen minutes. You can add honey to sweeten the tea if you desire, and feel free to drink this tea freely to soothe frazzled nerves.

Medicinal Uses

Burdock – Used medicinally to treat colds and flu, relieve joint pain and gout, bladder infections, digestive complaints, skin conditions like psoriasis and acne, and reduce bloat and kill germs.

Chamomile – Used medicinally for insomnia, muscle spasms, treatment of wounds and ulcers, digestive disorders, relief inflammation, and arthritis pain, and the symptoms of colds and nasal allergies.

Elderberry – Used medicinally to treat the flu and the common cold, leg and back pain, sinus conditions, chronic fatigue syndrome, and nerve pain.

Fennel – Used medicinally to treat bloating and water retention, acne, indigestion and constipation, and nasal and chest congestion.

Ginger – Used medicinally to aid in digestion, reduce nausea, and fight the symptoms of the flu and the common cold.

Raspberry – Used medicinally to relieve digestive disorders and diarrhea, relieve symptoms of the flu and the common cold, ease infections of the airways, and assist with heart problems.

Tila (Linden) – Used medicinally to induce sweating in people with fevers, relieve coughs and other throat irritations, reduce nasal congestion, and soothe nerves and high blood pressure.

Chapter 2: Scientific Studies on Alkaline Diet

Livelihood on Earth is based on the pH levels required in and around living cells and organisms. The human body requires a balanced pH level of approx. 7.4 with a slightly alkaline pH range between 7.35 and 7.45 to survive. Incredibly, the soils' pH level that was used to grow the plant foods we eat also has a noticeable effect on the mineral composition of the meals.

Studies showed that the ideal soil pH that will allow for essential nutrients is between 6 and 7. Plants planted in acidic soil with a pH level below the value of 6 may have reduced magnesium and calcium, and the ground with a pH level above seven can grow plants free of copper, manganese, zinc, and iron.

As we age, the muscles in the body experience a loss of muscle mass, which puts us at risk of falls and fractures. A three-year study considered a potassium-rich diet with foods like fruits and vegetables found that such a diet preserves muscle mass in older adults. A diet that corrects acidosis in the body can help us retain muscle mass in conditions with a loss of muscle mass such as trauma, kidney failure, diabetic ketosis, sepsis, and chronic obstructive pulmonary disease.

Alkaline supplement and growth hormone chronic forms of metabolic acidosis in young adults, such as renal tubular acidosis, have been linked to reduced growth hormone levels. In this case, acidosis can be corrected with potassium citrate or bicarbonate, which significantly increases growth hormone and therefore improves growth. Previous studies have shown that the use of sufficient quantities of potassium bicarbonate in a diet to reduce the net daily load of acid in postmenopausal women has significantly increased growth hormone.

Alkaline Diet and Back Pain

Previous studies have shown that supplementing with alkaline minerals can help improve chronic low back pain. With the integration of alkaline metals, there was a significant increase in intracellular magnesium and the blood's pH level. When there is enough intracellular magnesium in the body, the enzyme systems work well, which activates vitamin D, which in turn improves low back pain.

Alkalinity and Chemotherapy

The pH strongly influences the effectiveness of the substances or agents used for chemotherapy. Different agents such as Adriamycin and epirubicin rely on an alkaline agent to be more productive. Other chemotherapeutic agents such as thiotepa, cisplatin, and mitomycin are cytotoxic if present in an acidic medium. Studies have shown that inducing metabolic alkalosis can improve treatment regimens that use furosemide, carb cab, and baking soda. Also, extracellular alkalinization with bicarbonate can significantly improve therapeutic efficacy.

Discussion

The human body can maintain a stable blood pH with the primary respiratory and renal mechanisms. The vast majority of the body's membranes require an acidic pH to aid the digestion of food. Previous studies have shown that an alkaline diet reduces the risk of developing certain diseases and offers significant health benefits.

Macronutrients

You must take care of your macronutrient needs. The only thing you need to keep in mind when developing the alkaline diet is that the number of macronutrients you are taking in your body can dictate how acidic or alkaline you will be, which is why you must choose the macronutrient it needs appropriately and, of course, based on your goals. Many of you have the goal of getting rid of a disease or merely staying healthy overall. This is excellent, but you need to keep in mind that following the alkaline diet is that you can't have too much protein as it can become very acidic. On the other hand, you cannot have zero proteins since protein is a requirement for your daily needs.

Lose Weight

If you are trying to lose weight, the alkaline diet could work for you. However, making sure to get enough micronutrients in the diet can be a little tricky. That said, let's talk about the macronutrient needs that will be asked of you when you follow the alkaline diet. Keep in mind that you won't get enough protein if you don't take care of it. It means that you must be extremely meticulous with the foods you are eating to get enough protein. Achieving weight loss with an alkaline diet may happen, but you must also make sure that you exercise enough in your daily routine to supplement your goals. Keep in mind that when your goal is to lose weight, you need to make sure your proteins are on the top. The reason your proteins need to be on the top is that proteins take more calories to digest, which means you will only burn calories by eating protein.

Reduce the Risk of Disease

When your goal is to reduce the number of conditions you may be attracting, you need to consider that you need to be more on the alkaline side to achieve this. This would mean that you cannot have as much protein as someone who is merely trying to lose weight. That said, let's talk about the macronutrient needs that will be asked of you when your goal is to reduce the risk of disease and better results. The first thing you need to make sure of when you follow the alkaline diet is that you have to start by eating the right foods that will allow you to remain salty.

As you know, proteins take a lot of energy to digest food, which is why a fair amount of protein in the diet will help you maintain the muscle mass you have while keeping your body very alkaline. You can also consider having alkaline water to improve chemical levels throughout the day further. Now, when you're trying to reduce your risk of disease, you can still have the calories you want. But ideally, you shouldn't go beyond the maintenance calories you need during the day if you overestimate it, increasing your chances of gaining weight and increasing your risk of disease.

Get Rid of Diseases

Now, if you are in an unfortunate situation where you are facing illness, there is still hope for you. Many personal experiences have shown that the alkaline diet has helped users get rid of cancer and help them with chemotherapy. Also, if you are facing hypertension or other diseases, the alkaline diet can help you get rid of those. Keep in mind that these claims come from personal experiences and are not supported by science. However, since many people claim to have gotten rid of the diseases using the alkaline diet, you may also want to try it. Now, when your goal is to get rid of the infection, the breakdown of macronutrients will be a little more different than both of these diets.

This would be the complete break for anyone who is trying to get rid of their diseases, keep in mind that 20% protein will only give you enough protein to maintain muscle mass. Our goal is to stay as alkaline as possible to get rid of diseases, which is why we are taking in the minimum amount of protein during the day to ensure that we keep our muscles intact and that we are strong.

Some Diet Tips

To switch to Dr. Sebi's diet plans, it will be best to make small changes in the beginning to your overall eating habits. Gradually, these small changes will prepare you mentally and emotionally.

Emotional and Mental Preparation

Eating is an essential part of our lives. It is important to provide everyday's energy and nutrition requirements for our body. The types of foods and substances we eat every day become our habits, and these habits can last for our lifetime if we do not try to mind them.

Usually, all of these habits can be extremely hard to change or stop. Moreover, the influence of our friends, family, and colleagues makes it hard to change our daily habits. For example, you can't deny a piece of cake and other junk foods if it is a birthday party at your own home.

Therefore, before you rush to start with Dr. Sebi's diet, you should make a plan about changing your diet habits. A start without a proper plan and understanding may fail due to a lack of preparation. It will be best to discuss and reveal your plans to all the people you interact with within your regular life.

Drink More Water

Water is essential for our bodies. It is well known that around 75% of our body is water, and we can't survive even for three days without water.

Drinking more water cleanses our bodies and maintains our healthy brain and body functions. Among Dr. Sebi's products, Bromide Plus Powder has natural herbs like Bladderwrack that induce laxative effects and promote urination to help remove toxins. Drinking more water will replenish this lost water and will keep you hydrated.

It is recommended to drink up to one gallon of spring water every day. Springwater is recommended because it is alkaline in nature.

Add Whole Foods to Your Diet

You should add more whole foods to your existing diet, whether it is your favorite fruit or a fresh plate of fish. The basic idea is to consume whole foods to replace packaged foods that are full of additives. Cutting off these additives from your diet will help you later in your plans.

Also, note that refined sugar is highly addictive, and it can cause you to have food cravings.

Learn Basic Recipes

You should start with the foods which you already eat as a part of your diet. It doesn't matter if you are taking a vegan diet or not but make sure that you are not using any processed meals. It will be best to cook your own food, which means homemade food is recommended.

After you leave the processed food completely and homemade food becomes your daily habit, you are on the right path to regain health, and your next steps will bring you totally towards the right diet.

Read Ingredient Labels

For some people, it won't be easy to quit the processed food at once. But before you consume such foods, be sure to check the food ingredient labels. This will help to stay alert about what you are eating or drinking.

In the beginning, as you are not eating a strict diet, checking the labels will make your nutrition-conscious, and it will help you in changing your habits as you will progress.

Later, when you switch to a proper strict diet plan, you will still be conscious about your nutrition if you go astray from it.

Snacks

Snacks are very addictive. It becomes your compulsive habit, and you eat and eat without watching the nutrition status. Many people like to have snacks now and then, but instead of eating chips, why not try a mixture of walnuts, raisins, and other dried fruits? These dry fruits will replace processed snacks and will provide you with the proper nutrition.

Sebi Approved Meal Ideas

Dr. Sebi approved many meal ideas for better nutrition. Here are a few easy recipes that you can try at your home. They all use a minimal amount of ingredients and provide you with the proper nutrition while saving you from acidic foods.

4

Chapter 3: Dr. Sebi Approved Alkaline Foods

Dr. Sebi approved foods that are solely Alkaline foods are natural nutrients and beneficial to the general health of anyone who decides to follow them. However, you should know that these foods aren't supposed to substitute medications and medical advice. This notion is widespread among proponents of this diet. They always emphasize the fact that they aren't medical practitioners, just dieticians and nutritional consultants who suggest health nutrition as taught by Dr. Sebi.

Dr. Sebi Approved List of Foods

- **Vegetables:** amaranth, Nopales, Kale, Okra, Watercress, Squash, Onions, Mushrooms, Izote, Lettuce, Purslane, Zucchini, Wild Arugula, Tomatillo, Olives, Turnip greens, Sea vegetables, avocado, bell pepper, cucumber, chayote, dandelion, garbanzo beans.
    -
- **Fruits:** apples, Prickly Pear, Mango, Currants, Cantaloupe, Berries, Dates, Figs, Limes, Banana, Elderberries, Grape, Plums, Melons, Orange, Raisins (seeded), Tamarind, Papaya, Melon, Pears, Prunes, Soft jelly coconuts.
    -

- **Grains:** amaranth, fonio, wild rice, quinoa, spelt, Kamut, Tef, Rye.

- **Natural Herbal Teas:** Raspberry, Fennel, Chamomile, Ginger, Tila, Burdock, Elderberry.

- **Nuts and seeds:** this includes nuts and butter gotten from seeds. They include Brazil Nuts, Hemp Seeds, Raw sesame "Tahini" butter, Walnut, Raw Sesame Seeds.

- **Oils:** this category is divided into two, namely

- **Cookable oil:** this includes Sesame oil, Avocado Oil, Hemp Seed Oil, Grapeseed Oil.

- **Uncookable oil:** this includes olive oil and coconut oil. They are mostly drizzled on top of different recipes.

- **Spice and seasoning:** This category is subdivided into four groups.

- *Mild flavor:* spices in this category include Basil, Thyme, Tarragon, Savory, Oregano, Cloves, Bay Leaf, Dill, and Sweet Basil.
- *Salty flavor:* spices in this category include pure sea salt, Kelp, Dulse, Nori, Powdered Granulated Seaweed.
- *Pungent and spicy flavor:* spices in this category are Achiote, Sage, Habanero, African Bird Pepper, and Onion Powder.
- *Sweet flavor:* they are Pure Agave Syrup (from cactus) and Date Sugar.

Fundamentals Things to Recognize About Alkaline Diets

Alkaline diets are starting to gain recognition around the globe as essential persons and celebrities now come out openly to declare their unflinching support for this diet. Albeit, proponents of alkaline diets, claim that it is highly nutritional and equally beneficial to blood pH, this stand hasn't been accepted by science. These are the fundamental things you should know about this diet.

Foods Do Not Alter the PH Levels of Your Blood

Usually, having a blood pH of around 7.4 is healthy, and your body will most likely maintain these levels unless the vital organs, that is, the kidneys and lungs, which maintain these levels, get affected. Note that the consumption of alkaline foods doesn't affect the blood pH; instead, it only controls the acids close to your cells and determines if your urine is highly acidic or basic. You are only required to remain healthy and eat alkaline foods that are naturally healthy.

Alkaline Foods and Weight Loss

Alkaline foods encourage the consumption of solely plant foods and kicks against eating animal protein and refined foods. Although these foods are low-fats and promote weight loss, it is still required that you remain disciplined about your food consumption and active physically to achieve weight loss. Finally, it is an undisputed fact that alkaline foods are rich in various nutrients, and they help achieve optimal health. However, if you are in search of pH regulating foods, you should see a doctor because no food recipe can do this.

Foods to Avoid on the Alkaline Diet

The importance of food as a primary determinant of a person's wellness cannot be underemphasized. This is the reason behind alkaline diets.

Are you wondering why some food is terrible even when they are tasty, and you feel like you can't do without them? Are you curious about the benefits of foods apart from the sweet taste they have? Your answer is here as this topic will guide you on some commonly consumed foods and the reason why they are deemed unhealthy by Dr. Sebi.

These foods include:

MEAT: This includes meats rich in animal protein such as chicken, turkey, and red beef.

First, you should know that one of the reasons why this food is deemed unhealthy by Dr. Sebi is because of its high acidity. The continuous consumption of this food allows the development of excessive uric acids. This affects the blood and is detrimental to joint and tissue development. As a substitute for meat, you can consume plants like spirulina, which are highly rich in plant protein.

DAIRY PRODUCTS: This food, which includes milk and cheese, is highly toxic once digested because of its high acidity.

Dairy products are rich in two nutrients. That is phosphorus and calcium. However, while the required range of these nutrients should be 1:2.5, the ratio in dairy products is 1:1.27; that is, the level of phosphorus added to the body when dairy products are consumed is lesser than the calcium added which makes its consumption unhealthy to the body.

When our body lacks calcium, it becomes more acidic, and this is detrimental to organs, tissues, and bones.

An alternative to dairy products is nut milk, which is more nutritious and less toxic to dairy products.

GRAINS: Grains that are not gluten-free are unhealthy and unsuitable for alkaline diets. Apart from the fact that they are highly acidic, they also promote indigestion and cause skin inflammation.

Gluten-free alternatives include Rye, Quinoa, Spelt, etc. Although these plants can still be classified as acidic ones, they are less detrimental to general well-being than glutinous grains.

Hence, eating an exclusive grain alkaline diet is not advisable. Consuming grains in small quantities is best for maximum health benefits.

EGGS: This food also falls under harmful foods because they are highly rich in purine, which forms uric acid.

Hence, the consumption of eggs should be reduced and should be consumed with the right amount of alkaline diets.

LEGUMES: First, you should know that legumes fall under this list because they have low acidity. This food, because of its numerous health benefits, cannot be entirely ignored.

Hence, the consumption of small quantities of legumes can be included in the alkaline diet. They are useful in regulating blood sugar and also provide the body with energy.

So, if you can overlook the acidity factor, this legume is beneficial to you.

NUTS: While some nuts are highly alkaline and beneficial to health, some are detrimental.

Hence, reducing the amount of nuts you eat is advised. But they shouldn't be entirely neglected.

ALCOHOL: The consumption of alcohol is prohibited from alkaline diets. This is because, after digestion, alcohol leaves the body highly acidic and kills nutrients such as magnesium that help the body to remain alkaline.

Also, alcohol has adverse effects on our stomach, and it is detrimental to our stomach due to its high acidity.

COFFEE: This food has a high concentration of acids, and it also requires the removal of essential nutrients from the body to detoxify body.

Every single coffee flavor has high acidity. And no coffee flavor is advised. If you plan to make coffee, take an alkaline coffee.

PROCESSED SUGAR: The consumption of processed sugar is unacceptable for alkaline diets. This is because processed sugar and anything with processed sugar is highly toxic because of their high acidity.

Hence, the consumption of candy, chocolates, white bread, muffins, and other sugar-related foods isn't acceptable and should be avoided for an effective alkaline diet.

One leading cause of acidity in several humans is sugar consumption. It also promotes cravings and addiction, leading to increased stress in the body.

If you love to consume sweet things, try adding pure agave syrup or date sugar instead because they leave your diet sweet, and prevent high acidity.

5

Chapter 4: Intermittent Fasting

The First Week

Intermittent fasting in the first week, you are merely going to familiarize yourself with the window. It comprises the early seven days of starting your intermittent fasting exercise.

Tasks

- Select your preferred eight-hour eating window. Remember, sleep is part of your fasting window.
- Do not change the type of food you eat or consume. This week is about getting accustomed to the eating window.
- Do not take part in any exercise. If it is your first time of fasting, exercise will most certainly spike hunger, making discipline a tough task. Only be focused on staying within your window.
- Practice the 16:8 method of fasting from Monday to Friday and have the weekend off.

The Second Week

If you were able to stick to the tasks listed the first week, move on to the functions listed below. For the second week, sleep will be addressed, and we continue to practice the 16:8 eating method. Many benefits come with sleeping, which is why it is included this week.

Tasks

- Does it need to be changed? Does it fit with your daily schedule? If the answer is yes, continue to practice this fasting window from Monday to Friday. If not, choose a new eating window and repeat week 1. You are already conversant with the fasting system.
- Make sure it becomes a routine for you.
- Have a better sleep.
- Feel free to do some light exercise if you have itchy feet! Nevertheless, I would still advise no use if you are battling with a hunger to allow you to adapt fully to your eating window. Before you go into the practice, you have to determine which one is the best for you to avoid unnecessary zapping of energy.
- Once more, do not entirely change the type of food you eat. You can add a few additions to your eating circle, but do not change totally.

The Third Week

This week, exercise will be added. You have perhaps been hankering to burn some calories if you haven't started exercising at all!

Tasks

- Go through your eating window. Is it still working? Do you need to change it to help you be more devoted to the exercise? If the window is okay, continue with your current window Monday to Friday fasting. If not, choose a new window and start from week 1. Starting again doesn't mean you are failing in your quest for intermittent fasting. You are only getting to know which one is the best for you.
- Add suitable workout training based on your level of ability. Create a workout schedule to complete two three times this week. Remember to

always consult an appropriate professional before going through any diet or exercise plan.

- Continue to practice your chosen tips for sleep quality from the last week.
- Start to cut back on sugar. The person himself determines this task. Most people certainly know where they need to start.

The Fourth Week

By the fourth week, you should have your perfect eating window in place. If you are still finding it hard to have a stable eating window, I strongly advise you to see professionals in this field.

Tasks

- Continue with your selected eating window, which is from Monday to Friday.
- Add some of the foods that have magnesium and potassium in them to your meal.
- Look for appropriate dessert options to help keep you healthy! The logic here is to find keto desserts as they will be low in carbohydrates and high in fat. Recollect that fat gives less insulin and will assist your body to switch to using fat for energy. Do not rely on the "low fat" agenda.
- Have a better sleep (preferably with sunlight).
- Continue to remove sugar from your meals.

The first 30 days of 16:8 aren't drastic, as you can see. I have not outlined whether to give up pasta, potato, or even sweet treats. You will spend your first 30 days making positive changes, and producing great results to keep you motivated. The key to success in the long term lies in how you start. As a beginner, I advise against rushing forward, even though I know how desperate you are for results. Initially, the number one reason people give up is by trying too much, too fast. Often, we've been overweight or obese for 5-20 years. It is unreasonable to expect in the blink of an eye that you will change life-long patterns and lack discipline!

6

Chapter 5: The Six Stages of Intracellular Interaction in the Body

Intermittent fasting is not a hack for weight loss that bodybuilders use to maintain muscle mass and lose fat quickly. Intermittent fasting is more than that - it is a diet plan that was developed through the evolution of science and the study of human body metabolism.

The fasting program informs the body to return to its best condition and be highly effective in its operations. This process of body conditioning prompts various bio-mineral and cellular interactions within the body, which subsequently creates a shift in body metabolism.

These interactions are what brought the stages of cell dynamics in the system. The stages include;

Stage 1: Ketosis

Stage 2: Autophagy

Stage 3: Growth hormone

Stage 4: Insulin reduction

Stage 5: Immune system cell rejuvenation

Stage 6: Re-feeding

This long process is what your body undergoes in order to become transformed. But we really need to know when these interactions usually take place. Timing is very important in our fasting, and understanding timing relative to the body's reactions is very vital in intermittent fasting. So, let's look at the stages and times at which each of them is expected to take place.

Stage 1 - Ketosis

Once your body stays for about 12 hours without food, it starts to burn fats already stored in the system. The liver uses some of these fats to produce ketones, under a state called ketosis.

These ketone bodies function as an alternative energy source for our body cells. These ketones help to prevent cell death and lower inflammation. It also promotes mental clarity. Within 18 hours of no food, your body starts to generate enough ketones as it enters into fat-burning mode. At this stage, you can easily measure the ketone level in your body.

Stage 2 - Autophagy

Twenty-four hours into the fasting, your body cells will start breaking down old components, including proteins that are associated with diseases like Alzheimer's. This stage is known as autophagy, a process for tissue and cell rejuvenation.

Autophagy helps to remove dead cells. Once your body stops initiating autophagy, it starts to experience difficult conditions like neurodegenerative diseases. This is one of the major causes of disease during old age. Calorie restriction with enough exercise during fasting increases autophagy in body tissues.

Stage 3 - Growth Hormone

Prolonging fasting or calorie restriction up to 48 hours triggers the release of growth hormone. The level of growth hormone rises five times compared to the time you started your fast.

Ketones and ghrelin, a hunger hormone, promote the secretion of growth hormones. This growth hormone plays important roles in the body such as healing of wounds, reduction of fat tissue accumulation, preservation of lean muscle mass, and cardiovascular health.

Stage 4 - Insulin Reduction

At this stage, your insulin level has dropped to the lowest point, making your body highly insulin sensitive. Drastic insulin reduction happens after about 54 hours of fast or restriction. This helps to reduce inflammation in the body and keep the body free from various chronic diseases.

Stage 5 - Immune Boost

Getting to 72 hours, old immune cells break down, and the body generates new immune cells. A good condition for anyone undergoing chemotherapy as it helps to preserve white blood cells.

Stage 6 - Re-feeding

The 5 stages make our body feel light and refreshed and prepare the body for any diet. At this stage, the body can easily adapt to any healthy eating lifestyle. Along with Dr. Sebi's diet, the body can become fully detoxed, and the liver completely cleansed.

High Protein Diet

A high protein diet includes a large quantity of protein and only a small quantity of carbohydrates. Food that is rich in protein helps a person feel full, reducing the need for more calorie intake. A high protein diet has been known to have an impressive impact on the appetite, the body's metabolic rate, and the body's composition. Protein diets produce certain hormones on the body that helps to feel full and satisfied. It reduces the production of the hormone ghrelin, which is also known as the hunger hormone.

Low-Calorie Diet

Contrary to many people's opinions, a low-calorie diet does not mean low on nutrients. It just means feeding your body with healthy foods that support your health and enhances weight loss. Low-calorie diets are a diet that reduces calorie intake to about 1200-1600 per day for men and 1000-1200 per day for women. Some people go on a very low-calorie diet, consuming only about 800 calories per day. But for effective weight loss without adverse effects, a low-calorie diet is advised against a deficient calorie diet. This is because a less extreme diet is easier to adhere to, and they tend to interrupt daily activities less. By eating a low-calorie diet, you create a calorie deficit that can ultimately lead to weight loss. The logic with a low-calorie diet is when you eat less calories than your body burns, the body results in burning the body's fat store to make up for the calorie shortfall.

Some good examples include oat, berries, eggs, chia seeds, cottage cheese, potatoes, lean meat, legumes, watermelon, tomatoes, walnut, soup, shakes, celery, arugula, radish, cucumber, grapefruits, wheat bran, mussels, lentils, etc.

Water

Drinking water has been known to help boost metabolism, which, in turn, helps to burn excess fat in the body. It is also known to be actively involved in cleaning the body of waste and act as an appetite suppressant. Studies have shown, drinking more water helps the body to stop retaining water, leading to a significant drop in the extra pound gotten from water weight. It is advised that water is taken before meals. Because it is an appetite suppressant, it will reduce the amount of food you eat. The average reduction in intake measures up to 75 calories when water is taken before a meal. You can imagine how many calories you will lose per day, week, month, or year if you decide to start taking water before each meal. Studies have shown that by replacing calorie-filled drinks with water, you tend to lose more weight. If you think water tastes boring, you can add lemon to the water as this has a good track record in enhancing weight loss. It is better to drink this water cold as the body has to work harder to warm the water up, thereby boosting metabolism.

For people who are strong and healthy enough, water fasting is also advised.

Fibre

It acts as a bulking agent to help form stools. On the other hand, soluble water mixes with water to form a viscous gel-like substance, which slows down how fast the stomach releases food into the gut and gives a feeling of fullness, thereby reducing the need for more food intake. Fibres are known to feed friendly bacteria in the gut. These bacteria contribute significantly to various aspects of health, of which weight management is one. Fibres make the stomach full, thereby stimulating the brain's center that tells us to stop eating. Besides, Some examples include beans, flax seeds, legumes, asparagus, Brussels sprouts, oats, berries, barley, brown rice, bran, spinach, carrots, green beans, banana, prunes, apple, peanuts, squash, guava, figs, kiwi, beets, etc.

Low-Fat Diet

Most of the body's excess weight comes from the abundance of fat deposits that are gotten from the consumption of calories the body doesn't need and also from the consumption of unhealthy food products. There are about four different types of fats: Saturated fats, monounsaturated fats, polyunsaturated fats, and Trans-fat. Saturated fats contain excess calories. They are found in meat, hotdogs, bacon, sausages, which add those additional fats the body doesn't need. Monounsaturated fats contribute greatly to weight loss as they contain fewer calories. They support healthy energy levels in the body. They are found in avocado, olives and olive oil, macadamia nuts. Polyunsaturated fat includes omega 3 and omega 6, which are good for the heart and healthy for the body.

Paleo Diet

It encourages healthy whole foods. With the paleo diet, you eat food that fills you up and makes you feel less hungry throughout the day, reducing unnecessary intake of additional calories. It also helps to reduce appetite and cut down on the rate at which we eat.

7

Chapter 6: Dr. Sebi Approved Herbs and Food Items

Dr. Sebi Diet Rules

You must observe these main guidelines, according to Dr. Sebi's dietary guide:

Rule 1. You have to consume foods specified in the nutritional manual.

Rule 2. Drink 1 gallon (3.8 liters) of water daily.

Rule 3. Take the supplements by Dr. Sebi one hour before taking medications.

Rule 4. No animal products are allowed.

Rule 5. Alcohol is not allowed.

Rule 6. Avoid wheat goods, and use only the "natural grains" specified in the guide.

Rule 7. Avoid using a microwave to keep the food from being poisoned.

Rule 8. Eliminate fruits that are canned or seedless.

There are no clear rules on the nutrients. This diet is low in protein, though, as it excludes beans, lentils, and meat, and soy foods. Protein is an essential effective nutrient for strong muscles, skin, and joints.

In fact, you're supposed to purchase cell food items from Dr. Sebi, which are supplements that aim to clean the body and nourish the cells.

It is advised to buy the "all-inclusive" bundle, which contains 20 separate items promising to cleanse up and rebuild the whole body at the quickest possible pace.

Besides this, there are no clear guidelines for the supplements. Instead, you can order some medication that fits your health issues.

The "Bio Ferro" pills, for example, promise to cure liver issues, cleanse the blood, improve immunity, encourage weight loss, aid digestion disorders and enhance general well-being.

Additionally, the products do not include a full list of nutrients or their proportions, rendering it impossible to determine whether they can fulfill the everyday requirements.

Summary

Dr. Sebi's diet has eight main rules to fulfill. They concentrate mainly on eliminating animal products, ultra-processed food, and taking the patented supplements.

What Does It Mean to Alkalize the Body?

An alkaline diet is focused on the idea that the food you consume regulates the body's pH. Because the products that our body utilizes leave behind metabolic waste, the theory is that the waste will have a pH that ranges from alkaline to acidic.

In various areas, the human body has varying pH ratios, with organs such as the stomach becoming more acidic, whereas blood becomes more alkaline. One of the body products that is specifically influenced by the foods we consume is pee, which is a sensor in the blood to regulate pH.

The larger group of "alkaline diets" is focused on the topic of metabolic waste, and one of those is the Dr. Sebi diet. They are strong enough to promote consuming healthy plant-based foods. However, there is no study behind alkalizing the body, and the arguments made are not backed by evidence.

Dr. Sebi Approved Herbs List

- Anamu/Guinea Hen Weed: Whole Herb
- Arnica: Root, Flower
- Basil: Leaf, Essential Oil
- Bay leaves: Leaf
- Bladderwrack: Whole Herb
- Blue Vervain: Leaf, Flower
- Bugleweed: Aerial parts
- Burdock: Root
- Catnip: Aerial Parts
- Cancansa/Cansasa/Red Willow Bark: Bark
- Cannabis (Marijuana/Hemp): Flower, leaf, seed, stem
- Capadula: Bark, Root
- Cardo Santo/Blessed Thistle/Holy Thistle: Aerial Part
- Cascara Sagrada/Sacred Bark: Bark
- Cayenne/African Bird Pepper: Fruit
- Centaury/Star Thistle/Knapweed: Flowering Aerial Parts
- Chamomile: Flower, Leaf
- Chaparro Amargo: Leaf, Branch
- Chickweed: Whole Herb
- Clove: Undeveloped Flower Bud
- Cocolmeca: Root
- Condurango: Vine, Bark
- Contribo/Birthwort: Root, Aerial Part
- Cordoncillo Negro: Bark
- Cuachalalate: Bark
- Dandelion: Root, Leaf (Mainly root used as medicine)

- Drago/Dracaeana Draco/Dragon Tree: Leaf, Bark
- Elderberry: Berry, Flower
- Eucalyptus: Leaf
- Eyebright: Aerial Parts
- Fennel: Seed
- Feverfew/Santa Maria: Whole Plant, Root, Flowering & Fruiting
- Flor de Manita/Hand Flower Tree: Flower
- Ginger: Root
- Guaco/Mikania: Root
- Governadora/Chaparral: Leaf/Flower
- Hoodia Gordonii/Kalahari Cactus: Fleshy part of the stem
- Hombre Grande/Quassia/Bitter Wood: Bark
- Hortensia/Hydrangea: Dried Rhizome, Root
- Huereque/Wereke: Root
- Iboga: Root Bark
- Kalawalla: Rhizome, Frond, Leaf
- Kinkeliba/Seh Haw: Leaf, Root, and Bark
- Lavender: Flower, Leaves
- Lemon Verbena: Leaves, Flowering Top
- Lily of the Valley: Flower
- Linden: Flower
- Lirio/Lily: Flower, Bulb, Leaf
- Locust: Bark
- Lupulo/Hops: Flower
- Manzo: Root, Rhizome, Leaf
- Marula: Bark, Fruit, Leaf, Kernel, Nut
- Milk Thistle: Seed
- Mullein/Gordolobo: Flower, leaf, seed, stem
- Myrrh: Resin
- Nopal: Cactus
- Oak Bark / Encino: Bark
- Ortiga/Stinging Nettle: Leaf
- Pavana/Croton: Seed

- Pao Periera: Bark, Stem
- Palo Mulato: Bark
- Peony: Root, Root Bark
- Pinguicula/Butterwort: Leaf
- Prodigiosa/Bricklebush/Leaf of Life: Leaf
- Prunella Vulgaris / Self-Heal: Whole Herb
- Purslane/Verdolaga: Leaf, Young Shoot, Stem
- Red Clover: Flower
- Red Raspberry: Leaf
- Rhubarb: Root
- Salsify/Goatsbeard/Oyster Plant: Root, Leaves, Flower, Seed, Young Stem
- San Pedro Cactus: Whole Herb
- Santa Maria/Sage: Leaf
- Sapo/Saponaire/Hierba del Sapo/Mexican Thistle: Whole Herb
- Sarsaparilla: Root
- Sea Moss: Seaweed
- Sempervivum/Houseleek: Leaf, Leaf Sap
- Sensitiva/Shameplant/Dead and Wake: Dried Whole Plant, Root, Leaf, Seed
- Senecio/Groundsel/Ragwort: Whole Herb
- Soursop: Leaf
- Shepherd's Purse: Whole Herb
- Shiny Bush Plant/Pepper Elder: Root, Aerial Part
- Tila/Linden: Flower
- Tronadora: Leaf, Stem
- Turnera/Damiana: Leaf
- Valeriana/Valerian: Root
- Yarrow/Queen Anne's lace: Aerial Part, Essential Oil
- Yellowdock: Root
- Yohimbe: Whole Herb

Dr. Sebi Approved Food Items from each Food Groups

Dr. Sebi Vegetable List

As for all his electrical products, Dr. Sebi claimed that people could consume products other than GMOs. That involves fruits and vegetables rendered seedless or modified to produce more minerals and vitamins than naturally they do. Dr. Sebi's vegetable list is extensive and varied, with many choices for making multiple diverse meals. This list contains:

- Arame
- Amaranth
- Bell Pepper
- Avocado
- Cherry and Plum Tomato
- Chayote
- Cucumber
- Dulse
- Dandelion Greens
- Hijiki
- Garbanzo Beans
- Kale
- Izote flower and leaf
- Mushrooms except for Shitake
- Lettuce except for iceberg
- Nori
- Okra
- Nopales
- Olives
- Purslane Verdolaga
- Tomatillo
- Onions
- Sea Vegetables
- Squash
- Turnip Greens

- Wakame
- Watercress
- Zucchini
- Wild Arugula

Dr. Sebi Fruit List

While the list of vegetables is lengthy, the list of fruits is very restricted, and certain varieties of fruits are not allowed for the consumption when on a diet by Dr. Sebi. However, the selection of fruits is still providing a broad range of choices to diet followers. For example, on Dr. Sebi's food list, all kinds of berries are permitted besides cranberries, which is a fruit made by man. The list also includes:

- Bananas
- Berries
- Apples
- Currants
- Dates
- Figs
- Cantaloupe
- Cherries
- Grapes
- Limes
- Mango
- Prunes
- Raisins
- Soft Jelly Coconuts
- Melons
- Peaches
- Pears
- Plums
- Prickly Pear

- Sour soups
- Orange
- Papayas
- Tamarind

Dr. Sebi Food List Spices and Seasonings

- Bay Leaf
- Cayenne
- Cloves
- Achiote
- Basil
- Dill
- Oregano
- Habanero
- Powdered Granulated Seaweed
- Onion Powder
- Tarragon
- Thyme
- Pure Sea Salt
- Sweet Basil
- Sage
- Savory

Alkaline Grains

- Kamut
- Amaranth
- Fonio
- Quinoa
- Tef
- Rye
- Spelt

- Wild Rice

Alkaline Sugars and Sweeteners

- Coconut Sugar
- 100% Pure Agave Syrup from cactus
- Date Sugar from dried dates

Dr. Sebi Herbal Teas

- Elderberry
- Ginger
- Red Raspberry
- Burdock
- Chamomile
- Fennel
- Tila

Seeds and Nuts

- Walnuts
- Brazil Nuts
- Hemp seeds
- Raw Sesame Seeds

Oils

- Olive Oil
- Coconut Oil
- Grapeseed Oil
- Sesame Oil
- Hempseed Oil
- Avocado Oil

8

Chapter 7: Dr. Sebi; A Man Who Cures All Diseases

Impotence of Erection Dysfunction

Dr. Sebi maintains that the excess fat build-up in the body leads to clogging of the penis and prostate gland. The renowned doctor recalled being healed of his impotence after fasting for 29 days. With proper fasting, the body rids itself of excess triglycerides, calcification, cholesterol, and the rest. Infertility happens when the orifice of the penis gets clogged, fasting will reopen this orifice by draining the plaque clogging the wet area.

Asthma
Dr. Sebi got out of his asthmatic condition due to fasting.

Arthritis
Dr. Sebi's mother had arthritis, which made him place her on 53 days fast. During this period, she was only allowed to consume water and a list of pre-approved food. After this fasting period, Dr. Sebi's mother was able to lift her arms above her head.

The Heart

Fasting allows for free passage of air into the blood, organs, and arteries. The Ph balance of the blood in the body is where healing takes place. The immune system study has revealed that harmful microbes, getting sick, and acquiring diseases is due to a deficiency in the blood. An acidic Ph level will strip the body of necessary nutrients and its ability to maintain a strong immune system.

During the cleansing and healing process, you must keep in mind that you will need more rest than ever. As your situation demands, you might experience a phase better known as a healing crisis, one where things get worse before they get better. This phase is fondly referred to as the "reversing disease" phase. Here, the body revisits every kind of pain, disease, or skin rash it has ever experienced before total healing takes place. Depending on how long your healing process is, Dr. Sebi has highlighted eight things on how your immune system can be boosted.

The Method

1. Fasting
2. Exercise
3. Eat
4. Sleep
5. Usha Village (or stress-relieving practices)
6. Refrain from consuming detrimental foods
7. A Gallon of Water a Day
8. Dr. Sebi Compounds

If you plan to pay a visit to Usha village for your healing, there is a need for you to have practiced the other methods contained on this list. This is in a bid to hasten your healing process.

In attempting to emphasize the importance of plant-inferred iron, Dr. Sebi made certain and significant statements. An individual rarely becomes ill if his iron level is up. If you have a disease, regardless of what kind of disease, you are anemic. Iron is the mineral that carries oxygen to the brain. Iron must have carbon, hydrogen, and oxygen (the CHO channel). Iron is the spark attachment of the human body. When you experience the ill deficiency of iron inadequacy, it presents you with many diseases. Iron touches off the body and is the main magnetic mineral on the planet. Iron is magnetic and attracts different minerals. Extract magnesium, zinc, gold, calcium, phosphorus, and so forth.

Sickle Cell Anemia

It is the deprivation of iron fluorine. Sickle cell anemia occurs when blood plasma is broken down by mucus into a sickle. The mucus membrane sinks into the plasma, into the cell itself, the cell breaks up and separates. By removing the lining, the cell unites again. To maintain this level, the patient must receive high doses of iron phosphate. It is not ferrous oxide.

Food with High Iron Content

Guaco is an African plant rich in iron.

Yellow Dock rich in iron.

Sarsaparilla is the highest substance of iron.

Burdock is rich in iron, fluorine, and potassium phosphate.

9

Chapter 8: Dealing With Herpes

Dr. Sebi developed five effective herbal products that have helped a lot of people to heal herpes. These natural products are what you need to cure herpes.

Below are the main ingredients contained in Dr. Sebi's products for herpes:
·AHP Zinc Powder
·Triphala
·Pure Extract Giloy Tablets
·Punarnavadi Mandoor
·AHP Silver Powder

Let us do a detailed analysis of the elements contained in these products.

AHP Zinc Powder

The term AHP stands for ayurvedically herbo purified. The purification of zinc is done with decoctions of natural herbs such as aloe vera to produce AHP zinc powder.AHP zinc power is of a better benefit than the usual zinc tablets you consume. AHP zinc powder is prepared from naturally occurring zinc, making it very easy for your body to absorb.

AHP zinc powder also has the main qualities of some of the herbs used in preparing it. Modern medicine also acknowledges the importance of zinc for herpes treatment, but it is better to use AHP zinc powder instead of zinc tablets.AHP zinc powder is safer and more effective in treating herpes.

Triphala

Triphala contains three outstanding herbal combinations. The three herbs that makeup Triphala are harad, amla, baheda.

These three herbs have not only been acknowledged for their potency by Dr. Sebi, but other medical experts have conducted research on these three great herbs and praised theirefficacy.

This herbal combination is a good one that can be taken by both healthy people and people infected with the herpes virus.

This herbal combination can clean the unwanted materials and toxins in your bodyand help purify your blood and many organs in your body.

Dr. Sebi didn't only administer this herbal combination to his patients, but he also took it daily for optimal health and longevity.

Pure Extract Giloy Tablets

Pure extract giloy tablets are produced manually from the extracts of the best quality giloy.

Giloy is the perfect herb to improve your immunity and fight sexually transmitted diseases (STDs)

Dr. Sebi himself was a big fan of giloy, and now, modern medical experts have accepted that giloy can help your body fight off many diseases and improve health.

Punarnavadi Mandoor

Punarnavadi mandoor is not an herb purified mineral, but a healthy her-bomineral created from the combination of herbs and mineral.Punarnavadi mandoor is an extraordinary combination of healthy minerals such as calcium, iron, and great herbs such as shunti, punarnava, alma, etc.This herbomineral combination works perfectly on the liver and helps to eliminate toxins in the liver.

Dr. Sebi administered this herbomineral combination to many of his patients, and the reason for this is that the liver's function was disrupted during infection, and punarnavadi mandoor is the perfect option to bring the liver function back to normal.

AHP Silver Powder

Ayurvedically herbo purified (AHP) is a process that involves purifying various minerals in herbal decoctions, making them useful for medication.

AHP ensures that the minerals maintain their excellent abilities and absorb the nutrition and qualities from the herbs, which they are purified into.

AHP powder is exceptionally helpful to your health, especially your nervous system. Dr. Sebi administered AHP silver powder to several of his patients with herpes, and the results were always good.

What makes AHP silver powder effective for herpes is that it works on your neurons, the very place where the herpes virus in your body uses as itshome and hiding place.

AHP silver powder works by sending silver nanoparticles into your neurons to eliminate and flush out the herpes virus in your neurons.

Curing Herpes With Dr. Debi Diet on a Budget

Dr. Sebi's way of curing herpes is a simple process, and that is to nourish and detoxify the body. With this process, if you are looking to get rid of herpes from your body on a budget, here are some of the things you need to do:

Herbs and Fasting

One of the first things you can do is fast during the detoxification period, where you are taking in the necessary herbs alongside iron. On many occasions, Dr. Sebi has highlighted the importance of iron when healing. This means that during this period, we can use the combination of green juices, water, and herbs for proper detoxification.

Herbs and the Alkaline Diet

Following the alkaline diet while following the herpes healing process is important. The alkaline diet is one where you consume vegetables and other essential meals with the restriction of meat and other starchy meals.

The ingestion of starch and meat is something Dr. Sebi has stressed as something we need to avoid when healing herpes. We also have a recipe list that you can follow to help you stay on the alkaline diet while curing your herpes.

This means that your body is cleansed of whatever might be fighting the healing process while you replenish the body and boost your immune system.

Overall Guide

·At this point, you would avoid cooked food as much as possible.

·You would also take out any acid-forming foods from your diet.

·Fast while you take water and herbs.

·Once you have completed your fast, you would need to take fruits and vegetables to improve the healing process.

·Once your herpes is gone, you would need to continue with the Dr. Sebi recipes for a while to keep you healthy and make the healing process a permanent one.

Herpes is curable, as we know, with all we have learned from Dr. Sebi, and it can be done on a budget as well. You do not need to spend a fortune to get this done, and all you have to do is follow the simple process highlighted here.

Dr. Sebi's Herbs for Curing Herpes

For Dr. Sebi's herbs for herpes to work effectively for you, you have to start with the cleansing herbs.

Below are some of the cleansing herbs you need to take:

Cleansing Herbs

·**Mullein:** Mullein helps to cleanse the lungs and to activate lymph circulation in your neck and chest.

·**Sarsaparilla root:**Sarsaparilla root helps to purify the blood and target herpes. Jamaican sarsaparilla root is highly recommended because it is a great source of iron, and it is good for healing. This herb contains smitilbin, phenolic compounds, triterpenes, sarsaparilloside, and parillin. It is a therapeutic herb that helps in detoxification and blood purification. This herb is also effective against genital herpes, coldsores, dermatitis, shingles, and autoimmune problems. It is also important for the treatment of cancer, especially breast cancer.

·**Dandelion:**Dandelion helps to cleanse the gallbladder and the kidneys. Dandelion is rich in iron and potassium. It is one of the common herbs that are important for the curing of different diseases. It helps with cleansing and detoxification of toxic substances in the body. Dandelion is used for the treatment of herpes, hypertension, HIV/AIDS, urinary tract infection, breast cancer, skin infection, and hypoglycemia.

·**Chaparral:**Chaparral helps to cleanse harmful heavy metals from your gallbladder and blood and also cleanse the lymphatic system.

·**Eucalyptus:**You can use eucalyptus to cleanse your skin through sauna or steam.

·Guaco Herb: Guaco heals wounds, cleanses the blood, promotes perspiration, increases urination, keeps your respiratory system healthy, and improves digestion. Guaco plant is an anti-septic, operative, anti-bacterial, tonic, depurative, hemostat, fungicide, cholagogue, febrifuge, and laxative. This plant contains a high content of iron, strengthens the immune system, and contains potassium phosphate that makes it effective against the herpes virus. It is also a fever reducer, and helps in removing defective mucus in the body.

·Cilantro: Cilantro helps to remove heavy and harmful metals from your cells, and this is essential to heal herpes because the herpes virus hides behind your cell walls.

·Burdock root: Burdock root helps to cleanse the lymphatic system and the liver.

·Elderberry: Elderberry helps to remove mucus from the lungs and upper respiratory system.

Revitalizing herbs are what can heal the herpes virus. Revitalizing herbs are herbs and oils that target the herpes virus specifically. It is important you take these revitalizing herbs after cleansing and detoxifying your body so that the herbs can completely clean your body.

Here are Dr. Sebi's herbs that can heal the herpes virus:

·Pao Pereira: Pao Pereira effectively helps to subdue the herpes virus, and it also inhibits the duplication of the herpes virus genome.This herb is an awesome herb to help to fight the herpes virus.

·Pau d'Arco: The chemical constituents contained in Pau d'Arco have shown in vitro anti-viral properties against HSV-1 and HSV-2, and other viruses such as poliovirus, influenza, and vesicular stomatitis virus.

·Oregano Essential Oil: Oregano essential oil is a great anti-viral that can suppress the herpes virus. It works best at ninety percent concentration.Apply essential oregano oil to your lower spine because your lower spine is the point where HSV-2 is dormant.You can also apply it to your genital area and under your tongue.

·Ginger Essential Oil: Ginger essential oil can kill the herpes virus on contact. But you should dilute the ginger essential oil with a carrier oil The ginger essential oil has the same effect as the oregano essential oil.

·Sea Salt Bath: Sea salt helps to absorb electrolysis through your skin during a herpes virus outbreak. To succeed, you need to add a cup or half a cup of sea salt into a tub filled with warm water and soak your skin in it for some time.Ensure that the sea salt dissolves completely.

·Holy Basil: Stress is one of the factors that can trigger a herpes outbreak through adrenal fatigue. Holy basil is an adaptogen that relieves adrenal fatigue and prevents the outbreak of herpes through stress.

·Conconsan Plant: This plant is an African plant. The highest concentration of potassium phosphate is embedded in it, which fights against the herpes virus.

- **Purslane:** This plant is grown yearly in cold climates. It grows up to about 45cm. It is loaded with a rich amount of iron components. It is reported that this plant is effective for the treatment of herpes simplex virus.
-
- **Kale:** Kale is a rich source of calcium, antioxidants, and anti-inflammatory components. It is also loaded with more lysine. Lysine is an amino acid that is essential in suppressing the herpes virus. Lysine helps to prevent the multiplication of the herpes simplex virus.
-
- **Blue Vervain:** This herb is therapeutic. It contains a vast amount of iron

and helps in combating herpes simplex virus.

- **Lams Quarters (Pigweed and Wild Spinach):** This plant is rich in iron, and it helps in boosting the immune system.

- **Yellow Dock:** Yellow dock contains a rich amount of iron, and it is a tonic. It is important for the treatment of different diseases such as sexually transmitted diseases, intestinal infections, arthritis, and more. It contains lysine, which hinders the multiplication and growth of viral cells in the body.

How to Extract Essential Oils for Herpes

There are numerous oils for herpes, and the one thing that we have to consider is the extraction process. The proper extraction of these oils from their natural sources is a delicate process that requires a lot of experience and the right materials. There are numerous methods of extracting essential oils, but we are going to cover the two most important techniques, which are steam distillation and cold pressing.

Steam Distillation

The process of steam distillation makes use of steam and pressure for the extraction process. This process is a simple one, but without the right expertise, it can go wrong. The raw materials are placed inside a cooking chamber made of stainless steel, and when the material is steamed, it is broken down, removing the volatile materials behind. When the steam is freed from the plant, it moves up the chamber in gaseous form through the connecting pipe, which goes into the condenser.

Once the condenser is cool, the gas goes back into liquid form, and this is the essential oil that can be collected from the surface of the water.

Cold Pressing

The cold pressing process extracts oils from the citrus' rind, and the seed's oil. This process requires heat but not as much heat as the steam distillation process with a maximum temperature of 120F for the process to go as planned.

The heated material is placed in a container where it is punctured by a device that rotates with thorns. Once puncturing is complete, the essential oils are released into a container below the puncturing region. These machines then make use of centrifugal force to separate the essential oil from the juice.

Both processes are essential, and it has to be done properly with the right level of information from experts who know a lot about the process; if not, a lot more harm than good can and will be done.

Chapter 9: Food that Contributes to Weight Loss

High Protein Diet

A high protein diet includes a large quantity of protein and only a small quantity of carbohydrates. Food that is rich in protein helps a person feels full, reducing the need for more calorie intake. A high protein diet has been known to have an impressive impact on the appetite, the body's metabolic rate, and the body's composition. Protein diets produce certain hormones on the body that helps to feel full and satisfied. It also reduces the production of the hormone ghrelin, which is also known as the hunger hormone. All these factors combined automatically leads to a natural reduction in food intake. A high protein diet also increases the number of calories you burn most, especially when combined with exercise. This helps to build lean muscle in the body, and they are renowned for their ability to burn excess calories in the body throughout the day. Studies have shown that it does this by boosting the metabolic rate by about a whopping 20-35%. This also promotes weight and fat loss. Daily intake of about 1.2-1.6 grams per kilogram of your weight of a high protein diet can promote fat loss.

Low–Calorie Diet

Contrary to many people's opinions, a low-calorie diet does not mean low on nutrients. It just means feeding your body with healthy foods that support your health and enhances weight loss. Low-calorie diets are a diet that reduces calorie intake to about 1200-1600 per day for men and 1000-1200 per day for women. Some people go on a very low-calorie diet, consuming only about 800 calories per day. But for effective weight loss without adverse effects, a low-calorie diet is advised against a deficient calorie diet. This is because a less extreme diet is easier to adhere to, and they tend to interrupt daily activities less. Though most low-calorie diets leave you feeling hungry and unfulfilled between meals, a good combination with a high protein diet will help resolve the issue. There is some low-calorie diet that can give you the feeling of fullness and satiety that you desire. By eating a low-calorie diet, you create a calorie deficit that can ultimately lead to weight loss. The logic with a low-calorie diet is when you eat less calories than your body burns, the body results in burning the body's fat store to make up for the calorie shortfall.

Water

Drinking water has been known to help boost metabolism, and this, in turn, helps to burn excess fat in the body. It is also known to be actively involved in cleaning the body of waste and act as an appetite suppressant. Studies have shown that drinking more water helps the body to stop retaining water, leading to a significant drop in the extra pound gotten from water weight. It is advised that water is taken before meals. Because it is an appetite suppressant, it will reduce the amount of food you eat. The average reduction in calories in intake measures up to 75 calories when water is taken before a meal. You can only imagine how many calories you will lose per day, week, month, or year if you decide to start taking water before each meal. Studies have shown that by replacing calorie-filled drinks with water, you tend to lose more weight. If you think water tastes boring, you can add lemon to the water has this has a good track record in helping to enhance weight loss. It is better to drink this water cold as the body has to work harder to warm the water up, thereby boosting metabolism. For people who are strong and healthy enough, water fasting is also advised. This means the intake of water alone without food for a while because the body does not have calories to feed on. It results in burning the fat deposit in the body to provide the body with energy.

Fibre

There are types of fibre, soluble fibre, and insoluble fibre. Insoluble fibre does not mix with water. It acts as a bulking agent to help form stools. Soluble water, on the other hand, mixes with water to form a viscous gel-like substance, which slows down how fast the stomach releases food into the gut and gives a feeling of fullness, thereby reducing the need for more food intake. Fibres are known to feed friendly bacteria in the gut. These bacteria contribute significantly to various aspects of the health of which weight management is one. Fibres make the stomach full, thereby stimulating the centre in the brain that tells us to stop eating. Besides, fibres are more slowly digested than other carbohydrates, which mean food stays in your stomach for a longer period of time, and you don't feel the need to eat often.

Some examples include beans, flax seeds, legumes, asparagus, Brussels sprouts, oats, berries, barley, brown rice, bran, spinach, carrots, green beans, banana, prunes, apple, peanuts, squash, guava, figs, kiwi, beets, etc.

Plant-Based Diet

Low-Fat Diet

Most of the excess weight of the body comes from the abundance of fat deposits that are gotten from the consumption of calories the body doesn't need and also from the consumption of unhealthy food products. There are about four different types of fats they include saturated fats, monounsaturated fats, polyunsaturated fats, and Trans-fat. Saturated fats contain excess calories. They are found in meat, hotdogs, bacon, sausages, which add those additional fats the body doesn't need. Monounsaturated fats contribute greatly to weight loss as they contain fewer calories. They support healthy energy levels in the body. They are found in avocado, olives and olive oil, macadamia nuts. Polyunsaturated fat includes omega 3 and omega 6, which are good for the heart and healthy for the body. They are found in salmon, flaxseed, coconut oil, etc. the trans-fats are the worst kind of fat. This is because they are the product of the hydrogenation of healthy oils, which makes it unhealthy for the body. By taking a low-fat diet, you cut down on the great number of calories that are found in fat diets. Studies have shown that the standard low-fat diet lowers your calorie intake by about 30% of the usual daily fat intake. Fats contain about 9 calories per gram, which is quite high compared to 4 calories per gram contained in protein. It is advised to eat boiled or baked foods instead of fried foods for a low-fat diet, chicken and turkey should be peeled skinless before they are eaten, cut down on fatty diaries it is better to go for skimmed milk, low-fat yogurt, and cheese. Opt for leafy greens and fruits. Mushroom, garlic, white fish, egg whites, sweet potatoes contain low fat.

Dash Diet

The sad news is many people have refused to choose the dash diet for weight control because of some misconceptions they have. Some of this misconception includes: dash diet is only for people with hypertension, it only focuses on low sodium and no salt intake, it is unapproachable and many other ones. But the truth is the health benefit of taking dash diets goes beyond weight loss, and it is worth a try. Most studies have shown that DASH dieting is about sustainability. This means the dietary control is focused on the diet you can maintain and keep up with.

11

Chapter 10: What are the Pathways of Detoxification in the Body?

Nowadays, there are various ways in which humans have exposed themselves to toxins. These toxins are unavoidable as we every day come in contact with pesticides, pollutions, or chemicals. Hence, you can encourage detoxifying the organs responsible for detoxification by inculcating the intake of alkaline herbs and vegetables to prevent damage to these organs. There are seven channels that help the body to remove toxins and waste.

Examples of these channels are:

- The Liver.
- The Colon (bowels).
- The Skin.
- The Kidney.
- The Lymphatic system
- The Lungs.
- The Blood.

The Liver: The liver is a fundamental part of your body's detoxification system because it is important for several bodily processes. It is regarded as the powerhouse of detoxification. As a result, the liver has to be extremely taking care of because the human has a liver. When the liver is healthy, you are definitely going to experience optimal health and the prevention of diseases.

The liver filters the blood circulating from the digestive tract before passage to the rest of the body. It helps our body break down nutrients, remove dangerous chemicals, heavy metals, alcohol, and drugs. It also helps metabolize fats, remove surplus cholesterol, and plays an important role in breaking down carbohydrates into water-soluble substances that can be excreted from the body through the kidneys.

To naturally detoxify the liver, eat plenty of antioxidant-rich food, alkaline foods, stop the intake of alcoholic drinks, and Dr. Sebi forbidden food.

The Colon (bowels): The colon is also an organ of waste removal that helps to remove faces. When your colon is healthy, it breaks down the plenty of nutrients you consume within a day and allows it to be eliminated via feces. The colon also reabsorbs water from foods that have undergone digestion and converts them into feces.

Healthy elimination should be about 1-2 times daily, but when it is less than this, the waste may recirculate, and this might put too much load on your colon. Hence, the need to take in more alkaline-based vegetables and fiber becomes necessary to properly make your colon function.

A colon that has problems is liable to allow the penetration of bacteria and toxic substances in the intestinal wall, which subsequently results in food allergies, celiac disease, diabetes, Irritable Bowel Syndrome as well as Crohn disease.

The Skin: The skin is regarded as the biggest organ of detoxification. The skin is important in the excretion of toxins and protects the body against viruses, bacteria, other chemicals, and fungi.

It is typically opened to toxic substances via the following: toiletries, cosmetics, household cleaners as well as other compounds that could get transferred into the blood.

Skin problems like redness of the skin, eczema, acne, and psoriasis occur as a result of inflammation gotten from unhealthy diets and other materials used on the skin.

The Kidneys: the Kidneys are important in producing and removing urine as waste. The kidney is also essential in filtering blood. Hydration (drinking enough water) is vital in keeping your kidney healthy. However, a dehydrated kidney might subsequently result in kidney abnormalities.

Also, individuals suffering from diabetes and high blood pressure are most at risk of having kidney problems.

You can maintain a healthy kidney, drink a lot of water, eat vegetables and fruits, stick to the Sebian diets, and try as much as possible to lose weight.

The Lymphatic system: the Lymphatic system helps protect the body from viruses, bacteria, and many other disease-causing organisms. The Lymphatic system also helps in the release of toxins.

The lymphatic system is composed of lymph vessels, lymph nodes, and lymph. Tonsils, adenoids, spleen, and thymus are all part of this system responsible for getting rid of toxins in the body.

The lymphatic system should always be kept healthy by ensuring you engage in proper exercise and other activities that ensure proper circulation of blood. You can also consume alkaline vegetables and fruits that are loaded with antioxidants.

The Lungs: the lungs help in filtering out carbon dioxide, fumes, mold, and other airborne toxic substances. The accumulation of toxic substances in the lung could destroy the respiratory system.

The Blood: It transports and transfers substances throughout the body. The blood also delivers essential vitamins and minerals to where they are needed in the body. Hence, the blood needs to be taken care of.

Conclusively, the organs necessary for detoxification should be placed under perfect care. However, you do not need to spend too much money buying drugs or supplements as you can get your detox pathways easily detoxified.

Chapter 11: Benefits of Dr. Sebi's Diet

For a healthy body, the alkaline and acid apportion must be adjusted, estimated by the body's pH level. PH esteems run from 0 to 14, and 7 is viewed as impartial. Any worth under seven is considered to be acidic. Pure nourishment, for example, meat and meat subsidiaries, pastries, and some improved drinks, as a rule, create an extraordinary measure of acid for the body. Acidosis, an instance of an elevated level of acidic in the circulation system and body cells, is the primary file for the ebb and flow of various diseases dispensing numerous individuals. Some health experts' reason that acidosis is liable for multiple people's underlying conditions these days.

The alkaline or alkaline diet, which regularly presents in our body, kills the body's significant level of acidic to accomplish harmony state. This is the primary capacity of the alkaline in the body. Be that as it may, the nearness of the alkaline in the body is immediately drained because of the elevated level of acidic substance it needs to kill, and there is deficient alkaline nourishment expended to renew the loss alkaline.

Good for a Healthy Body

To arrive at the base of the diseases, our frameworks' pH esteem must be kept up in a healthy state. Normally happening alkaline nourishments can enhance the lost alkaline levels in the body during the killing procedure. By keeping up a healthy alkaline diet, adequate alkaline measures are recharged in the framework in this manner, taking the body back to the transcendent alkaline state.

So, what are the approaches to incorporate an alkaline diet into our dietary patterns? The fundamental initial step is to diminish the measure of pure nourishment admission. As we know, these nourishments contain numerous synthetics, which are the guilty parties in expanding the acidic level in our body. The following stage is to eliminate the admission of meat and their subordinates and the measure of alcohol. The last advance is to build the rule of fresh foods grown from the ground, as they usually are high in alkalinity.

Oranges and lemons known for being acidic proselyte into alkaline after assimilation and consumed by the body is a decent alkaline diet. By and large, we should devour 75% of essential nutrients every day. The higher the measure of alkaline food we put into our framework, the more prominent the balance of the acidic condition in our body.

Reverse the Aging Process

Maturing is brought about by the development of acid squanders and the ensuing breakdown of substantial capacities. At the point when a body is too acidic, a condition called acidosis happens. Acidosis is, essentially, the over-worrying of oxidation frameworks and the breakdown of lipids. At the point when this happens, it discharges free radicals into the circulatory system. Free radicals are cells that assault cell dividers and films; executing the cell dividers and layers before at long last murdering the phones themselves. At the point when this happens, the apparent outcome is wrinkled, poor vision, age spots, awful memory, exhaustion, broken hormones; in short - untimely maturing. By expelling these acids, you can avert further harm to your cells and even invert the breakdown procedure.

Weight Loss

As advocated by Dr. Sebi, plant-based diets help for weight loss and general well-being of the body because they contain natural vegetables, nuts, grains, legumes, and fruits. Dr. Sebi's diet eliminates meat, processed food, and dairy, so it naturally helps you to lose weight.

Reduced Risk of Disease

While inflammation is one of the body's first lines of defense, indicating infection and diseases, chronic low-dose inflammation can also be bad to the body. In fact, the presence of chronic inflammation can result in many kinds of diseases such as diabetes, stroke, and even cancer. Thus, diets that are rich in fruits and vegetables are linked to reduced inflammation caused by oxidative stress. Studies that look into individuals consuming plant-based foods have 31% lower incidence for developing heart diseases and cancer than those who consume animal products.

The many restrictions of the Dr. Sebi Diet make it hard for some people to stick by it. Before you decide to give up because this diet demands a lot from you, below are helpful tips that you can follow to become successful.

- **Research about Dr. Sebi's methodology:** Following this diet has several rules you need to know. Before you adopt this diet, you need to do due diligence by reading information.
- **Download the nutritional guide:** Make sure that you download the nutritional guide that will serve as your guide when choosing ingredients to cook your Dr. Sebi Diet-approved meals. You can also use the nutritional guide to make your meal plans.
- **Prepare your weekly meal plan:** Making a weekly meal plan will not only organize your pantry but it will also allow you to think of delicious meals that will keep you inspired and motivated to continue following the diet. Planning your weekly meal plan will also help you know how much food you need to buy or stock in your pantry.
- **Plan your shopping trips:** Planning your shopping trips is especially important when following the diet. Schedule your shopping trips, especially if you need to buy your ingredients from different places. By organizing your shopping trips, you will be able to buy all the ingredients that you need to create delicious meals for the week.
- **Do fasting:** The diet is all about allowing your body to detoxify. To help with this process, you can also do fasting to jumpstart the detoxification of your body.

· **Find support:** Find like-minded people to give you the morale boost that you need while following the program. Look for groups within your community or online who also follow the diet.

Reduction of the Microbiome

The Microbiome is a term used to refer to microorganisms in your gut. Plant-based foods and foods rich in alkaline diet could reduce the microbiome in your gut, reducing the risk of you having an unwanted disease in your body.

Appetite Control

Eating a plant-based food containing fiber-rich foods such as beans and peas makes you feel full and satisfied compared to eating a meal that includes meat.

Strong and Healthy Immune System

Your immune system is weak because of disease and illness. A plant-based diet advocated by Dr. Sebi helps to strengthen the immune system and empowers your body to fight disease.

Reduce the Risk of Hypertension and Stroke

The healthy contents of plant-based diets help to reduce hypertension and your chances of having a stroke.

13

Chapter 12: Dr. Sebi Downside

Although Dr. Sebi's diet promises excellent results, however, there are some downsides to following the diet. Here are some of these disadvantages:

Lack of Essential Nutrients

Foods listed in Dr. Sebi's diet guide are excellent sources of vital nutrients, carefully selected to help the body stay healthy. However, following this strict alkaline diet may be at risk of a shortage of essential nutrients needed by the human body to function maximally. Although, this diet contains a list of supplements containing proprietary ingredients not listed in the products. This is a call for concern because one cannot determine what nutrients and quantity one should take them. This invariably makes it impossible to know if you are meeting the daily requirements of specific nutrients. And some of these nutrients include;

Protein Deficiency – This is a critical nutrient needed in the body. It is essential for muscle growth, the brain's health, production of hormones, bones' formation, secretion of enzymes, supports DNA, etc. According to the body's standard requirements to function and develop healthily, people above 19 years of age, either male or female, needs to ingest daily 56 grams and 46 grams.

And although some of the foods listed in this nutritional guide contain protein, they are not significant sources of this all-important nutrient. Some of these Dr. Sebi's approve foods containing protein include; hemp seeds which contain 31.7 grams of protein per 100 grams. One hundred grams of walnut would give you 16.8 grams of protein, which is similar to 100 grams of roasted chicken breast. So, for one to be able to meet up with the protein requirements of the body, it is advisable to consume a wide variety of foods rich in amino acids (proteins building blocks). But this is not possible because most of the other sources (excellent) of protein are in Dr. Sebi's forbidden food list. This includes; meat, lentils, beans and soy.

To meet up with the body's protein requirements daily, you would have to consume a particular, tiring, nearly impossible portions of food when following Dr. Sebi's diet. This will still leave the question of how much quantity and is it enough to meet the nutrient requirements every day.

Vitamin B-12 Deficiency – This may happen when a person does not consume enough of this vitamin, which could be another side effect of following Dr. Sebi's diet guide. This vitamin is part of the essential nutrients needed by the body. It functions to maintain the health of the nerves and also the blood cells. It is also critical to the formation of DNA. One of the excellent sources of vitamin B-12 is animal products which are prohibited by Dr. Sebi's diet.

The following symptoms are the result of vitamin B-12 deficiency, a worst case scenario of possible pernicious anemia, a condition that affects the body by hindering its ability to produce healthy and sufficient red blood cells. Other symptoms are depression, chronic tiredness, and tingling of the feet and hands. Although Dr. Sebi's herbal supplement promises to make up for the missing or inadequate nutrients in the food, because there is no quantitative measure listed on the supplement, one cannot know if one is consuming enough of the required nutrients.

Omega-3 Fatty Acids Deficiency – This nutrient is an essential part of the cell membrane. And it supports the health of the heart, brain and eyes. It is also a source of energy required by the body for carrying out daily activities, as well as boosting body's immune system. Although food like walnuts and hemp seeds found in Dr. Sebi's permitted list are plant sources of omega-3 acids, however, they are not sufficient.

According to research, omega-3 acids are easily absorbed by the body from animal products which are excellent nutrient sources. In order to ensure one is taking a sufficient quantity of omega-3 acids when following Dr. Sebi's diet or any vegan diet for that matter, it is advisable to take an omega-3 supplement daily. This will now lead us to the secondary side effect of following Dr. Sebi's diet.

Insufficient Calories and Negative Eating Habits

Following this diet plan could prove self-defeating because it could lead to negative or poor eating habits. This is as a result of insufficient calories associated with the diet. The diet encourages the use of supplements to balance the missing or inadequate nutrients in the plant-based diet. And supplements do not provide the body with calories. This will lead to under-eating, which could result in several mental, emotional and physical health issues.

The body needs 1,000 calories to function basically, and this is known as the resting metabolic rate. But when the body engages in physical activities, the body's calories could increase to about 2,000. So, consuming less would lead to slow metabolism, which will eventually lead to low energy. It could also lead to hair loss, constant hunger (which will lead to an unhealthy eating habit), infertility, sleep disorder, irritability, always feeling cold, constipation and anxiety.

Very Restrictive

Dr. Sebi's nutritional guide is highly restrictive as it forbids so much more food than it permits. It prohibits the consumption of all animal products and some plants, as we have seen earlier. It is so restrictive that it even forbids eating all seedless fruits and even some fruits with seeds (for example cherries).

Lack of Scientific Prove

This is the most important concern with following Dr. Sebi's diet. There is no scientific backing to all the promises of the diet plan. Dr. Sebi claims to change the body's pH (most importantly, the blood pH) through the foods we eat. However, some researches show that while the food we eat could slightly our urine pH temporarily, it cannot change the pH of the blood and that of the stomach (this is because it needs to maintain a certain level of acidity to carry out digestion). This is one of the reasons some people believe Dr. Sebi to either be a fraud or foolish.

Chapter 13: Dr. Sebi's Remedy Approach for Asthma and Other Diseases

Asthma and Cough

You may use KUNTA by Dr. Sebi

- 1 Teaspoonful Guaco
- ½ Teaspoonful Mullein Root
- 1Teaspoonful Hydrangea Root
- 1Teaspoonful Clove Plant

Preparing Techniques to Combine All Dr. Sebi Herbs

- Measure 1 Teaspoonful from each powder listed above for Asthma
- Pour the different quantitative powder inside a kettle and add 2 cups (500ml) of water.
- Put the Kettle on a heat source. At the boiling point, leave it for 8 – 12minus to boil and allow it to cool for some minutes to warm.
- Drink before a meal after meal at night before you sleep. Once-daily for 30 days.

Dr. Sebi technically applied close observation and regular supervision with the sufferers after administering appropriate therapy for prostate cancer.

He usually gave treatment to cure the fundamental cause, after he had gotten full health history from the sufferer.

The sufferer will be subjected to Thirty Days of Fast phase one detoxification and cleansing to degenerate tumor growth and fortify healthy cells.

Prostate and Breast Cancer

- Pavana (Croton tiglium)
- Cordoncillo negro or Matico (Piper aduncum)
- Kalawallia (Polypodium leucotomos)
- Burdock Root (Arctium lappa)
- Contribo (Aristolochia trilobata)
- Nettle Root
- Cupressus sempervirens

The enlisted herbal recipes for Cancer can be used separately through the infusion method of Dr. Sebi's herbal preparation.

Dr. Sebi Good To Do It Yourself

It is excellent to think about how to preserve your newly harvested plant after you have used enough of the cleanser to purify your body. As a result, the first thing of the powdered form.

Preparation of Powdered Form

Do the herbs' preparation separately when you have completed the processes, the preparation dosage can be determined.

- Harvest the herbs from the original source.
- Gently clean the herbs with pure water.
- Dice the herb into pieces
- Use clean Mortar and Pestle to pond it into a thin layer to expose the plant

tissue to hot-air, to facilitate quick and perfect dryness.

- Spread the herbs on foiled racks or aluminum trays and sundry or use hot air oven at 180 – 200oC. Make sure you turn the tray 90o at every 10 – 15minutes till it dries if you are using the hot-air oven.
- Grind the dried herb with a grinder to produce powdered form.

Cancer

To Combine All Dr. Sebi Herbs

- Measure 1 Teaspoonful from each powder listed above for Prostate Cancer.
- Pour the powder inside a kettle and add 3 cups (750ml) of water.
- Put the Kettle on a heat source. At the boiling point, leave it for 8 – 12minus to boil and allow it to cool for some minutes to warm.
- Drink at night only after a meal before you sleep.

Alternatively,

For Single Dr. Sebi's Herb

- Measure 1 Teaspoonful Cancer Powder
- Pour the powder inside a kettle and add 1 cups (250ml) of water.
- Put the Kettle on a heat source. At the boiling point, leave it for 8–12 mins to boil and allow it to cool for some minutes to warm.
- Drink at night only after a meal before you sleep.

You may also diffuse the powder in hot water.

Ready To Use Herbs

Many of the Dr. Sebi enlisted herbs for Cancer treatments are primarily available on the Amazon platform to be purchased.

Second Phase

You will need to follow all the nutritional requirements and reenergize your body system with the below herbs:

- Sarsaparilla Root
- Sea Mose (Iris moss)
- Pao Pereira
- Soursop
- Anamu also called Guinea Hen Weed.
- Sage

Prostatitis

The prostate often occurs in man's prostate gland. Prostate gland is situated under the urinary bladder and the branched ejaculatory duct that link with Urethra pass through it. When prostate is infected it enlarges and contracts the two ducts that passed through it, which prevents the passage of urine from the bladder through Urethra with severe pain or contraction.

The natural cleansing herbs to prevent or cure prostatitis by using Dr. Sebi.

28g of Dr. Sebi's Ready to Use Herbs Produce

- 1 Teaspoonful Blessed Thistle
- 1Teaspoonful Prodigiosa
- ½ Teaspoonful Cascara Sagrada Herb
- 1 Teaspoonful Rhubarb Root

100g of Dr. Sebi's Ready to Use Herbs Produce

- 1 Teaspoonful Cupressus sempervirens
- 1 Teaspoonful Burdock Root (Arctium lappa)

Preparing Techniques to Combine All Dr. Sebi Herbs

- Measure 1 Teaspoonful from each powder listed above for Prostatitis but take ½ Teaspoonful of Cascara Sagrada Herb.
- Pour the powder inside a kettle and add 2 cups (500ml) of water.
- Put the Kettle on a heat source. At the boiling point, leave it for 8 – 12minus to boil and allow it to cool for some minutes to warm.
- Drink at night only after a meal before you sleep.

Note: Confirm how many times you defecate before you increase the dosage. If you are frequently passing bowel once or twice daily, you do not need to increase the dose, but if you scarcely defecate once daily, you can start using the herbal medicine before a meal in the morning and after a meal at night.

Dr. Sebi Remedy Approach for Liver

Prepare for 30 day's Fast to ensure perfect detoxification, cleansing, and cellular fortification.

28g of Dr. Sebi's Ready to Use Herbs Produce

- 1 Tablespoon Bladderwrack Powder

100g of Dr. Sebi's Ready to Use Herbs Produce

- 1 Teaspoonful Sarsaparilla
- 1 Teaspoonful Yellow Dock Root
- 1 Teaspoonful Burdock Root (Arctium lappa)
- 1 Teaspoonful Nettle
- 1 Teaspoonful Elderberry Flower

Pack Dr. Sebi's Ready to Use Herbs Produce

- Two Packs of Sea Moss: Include it to your smoothie preparation.

Preparing Techniques to Combine All Dr. Sebi Herbs

- Measure 1 Teaspoonful from each powder listed above for Liver
- Pour the different quantitative powder inside a kettle and add 2¼ cups (562.5ml) of water.
- Put the Kettle on a heat source. At the boiling point, leave it for 8 – 12minus to boil and allow it to cool for some minutes to warm.
- Drink before a meal in the morning and after-meal at night before you sleep.

Dr. Sebi Remedy Approach For Indigestion and Pancreas Diseases
250g of Dr. Sebi's Ready to Use Herbs Produce

- 1 Teaspoonful Sage
- 1 Teaspoonful Prodigiosa
- 1 Teaspoonful Guaco

450g of Dr. Sebi's Ready to Use Herbs Produce

- 1 Teaspoonful Nopal
- 1 Teaspoonful Huereque

Preparing Techniques to Combine All Dr. Sebi Herbs

- Measure 1 Teaspoonful from each powder listed above for Liver
- Pour the different quantitative powder inside a kettle and add 2¼ cups (562.5ml) of water.
- Put the Kettle on a heat source, at the boiling point leave it for 8 – 12minus to boil and allow it to cool for some minutes to warm.
- Drink before a meal in the morning and after a meal at night before you sleep.

Dr. Sebi's Remedy Approach For Arthritis and Joint Inflammation
100g of Dr. Sebi's Ready to Use Herbs Produce

- 1 Teaspoonful Burdock Root (Arctium lappa)
- 1 Teaspoonful Sarsaparilla Root
- 1 Teaspoonful Elderberry Flower
- 1 Teaspoonful Chaparral
- 1 Teaspoonful Valerian Root

250g of Dr. Sebi's Ready to Use Herbs Produce

- 1 Teaspoonful Guaco

450g of Dr. Sebi's Ready to Use Herbs Produce

If, you are obese, diabetic and having high cholesterol you can add be below herbs to the above list.

- 1 Teaspoonful Huereque
- 1 Teaspoonful Nopal

Thermal Spring Water Bath

- You will need to make a thermal spring water bath before you sleep at night for 3 – 7days depends on the intensity of your arthritis.

Spring Water

Ensure you drink approximately 4liters of Spring Water daily.

Nutrition

Juice nutrition and vegetable foods should be taken during the use of cleaning for revitalization and microelement complements.

Preparing Techniques to Combine All Dr. Sebi Herbs

- Measure 1 Teaspoonful from each powder listed above for Arthritis
- Pour the different quantitative powder inside a kettle and add 3 cups

(750ml) of water.

- Put the Kettle on a heat source, at the boiling point leave it for 8 – 12minus to boil and allow it to cool for some minutes to warm.
- Drink before a meal in the morning and after-meal at night before you sleep.

NB: Suppose you are having high body resistance to the cleanser by not passing bowel or feeling congested after being taken the dosage prescription for 2 – 3 days without a significant effect. In that case you can add a half dose of the Cleansers.

To Increase the Dosage as following:

100g of Dr. Sebi's Ready to Use Herbs Produce

- 1½ Teaspoonful Burdock Root (Arctium lappa)
- 1½ Teaspoonful Sarsaparilla Root
- 1½ Teaspoonful Elderberry Flower
- 1½ Teaspoonful Chaparral
- 1½ Teaspoonful Valerian Root

250g of Dr. Sebi's Ready to Use Herbs Produce

- 1½ Teaspoonful Guaco

Preparing Techniques to Combine All Dr. Sebi Herbs

- Mix the whole 6 x 1 ½ = 9Teaspoonful powdered Cleansers together very well to achieve even distribution.
- Boil 9 Teaspoonful of the mixed with Three cups (750ml) of water for 8 to 12mins and cover it for few minutes to warm and drink half before a meal in the morning and repeat at night after a meal before you sleep.

Dr. Sebi's Remedy Approach For Hypertension
250g of Dr. Sebi's Ready to Use Herbs Produce

- 1 Teaspoonful Guaco

450g of Dr. Sebi's Ready to Use Herbs Produce

- 1 Teaspoonful Huereque
- 1 Teaspoonful Nopal

100g of Dr. Sebi's Ready to Use Herbs Produce

- 1 Teaspoonful Elderberry (Sambucus nigra L.)
- 1 Teaspoonful Burdock Root (Arctium lappa)

28g Of Dr. Sebi's Ready To Use Herbs Produce

- 1 Teaspoonful Rhubarb Root
- ¼ Teaspoonful Mullein Root

Preparing Techniques to Combine All Dr. Sebi Herbs

- Measure 1 Teaspoonful from each powder listed above for Hypertension
- Pour the different quantitative powder inside a kettle and add 3 cups (750ml) of water.
- Put the Kettle on a heat source, at the boiling point leave it for 8 – 12minus to boil and allow it to cool for some minutes to warm.
- Drink before a meal after meal at night before you sleep. Once–daily for 30 days.

If you want to be taken it in the morning, initially observe the number of times you defecate daily. If it is not more than once, then you can repeat the preparation in the morning before meal.

But if you are already defecting 3 – 4 times a day, do not repeat the treatment in the morning.

Dr. Sebi's Remedy Approach For Kidney
100g of Dr. Sebi's Ready to Use Herbs Produce

· 1 Teaspoonful Sarsaparilla
· 1 Teaspoonful Yellow Dock Root
· 1 Teaspoonful Burdock Root (Arctium lappa)
· 1 Teaspoonful Nettle
· 1 Teaspoonful Elderberry Flower

Pack Dr. Sebi's Ready to Use Herbs Produce

· Two Packs of Sea Moss: Include it in your smoothie preparation.

Preparing Techniques to Combine All Dr. Sebi Herbs

· Measure 1 Teaspoonful from each powder listed above for Kidney
· Pour the different quantitative powder inside a kettle and add 2¼ cups (562.5ml) of water.
· Put the Kettle on a heat source. At the boiling point, leave it for 8 – 12minus to boil and allow it to cool for some minutes to warm.
· Drink before a meal in the morning and after-meal at night before you sleep.

Chapter 14: Dr. Sebi's Immune and Respiratory Boosting Herbs

Out there, a lot of people are concerned about how they can build their immune system and keep their bodies healthy during this uncertain time. In the instance that we get sick, we want to know what we can do to combat the disease. Not everyone will subscribe to this school of thought, but the best thing to do in every situation is to trust the highest with the belief that whatever is meant to happen will eventually happen. However, it is also a good step of faith to prepare and equip ourselves with the right information and knowledge.

Things We Need In Order To Help Ourselves, Friends And Our Families During this Pandemic Include:

Foods and Herbs

To remain healthy and boost our immune systems, I will go over some herbs and foods that help to clear mucus from the respiratory system and help build the immune system.

Blue Vervain

This herb offers relief for liver and respiratory congestion; it lowers fever, calms the nerve, cleanses toxins, and serves as a general tonic that gives an overall feeling of well-being.

Bugleweed

This herb is great for the relief of breathing difficulty, coughs, colds, and respiratory illnesses. The herb also helps with bronchial congestion, the release of sinus, the relief of sore throat-related pain, and mucus discharge from the respiratory tract.

Cablote

Cablote is instrumental in the treatment of bacterial and viral infections in the upper respiratory system. The herb also helps to cleanse mucus in the upper respiratory system. Cablote is a favorite natural remedy amongst the indigenous people of Amazon as well as Central and South American health practitioners. It is mostly used for upper respiratory infections. It can also reduce fever, cure coughs as well as provide antibacterial and antiviral actions.

Cordoncillo Negro

This herb is majorly used to treat pneumonia, bronchitis, coughs, flu, cold, and other respiratory problems.

Elderberry

Personally, elderberry is one of my favorites. It helps to remove mucus from the lungs and upper respiratory system. The herb also helps with flu, cold, cough, viral, and bacterial infections. Additionally, it helps to build the immune system. I recommend that everyone should always have this herb at home.

Eucalyptus

This is another great herb that is often overlooked. It is majorly used for the treatment of congestion, asthma, sore throats, colds, coughs, and respiratory disorders.

You can be relieved of cough and congestion by rubbing eucalyptus ointment or oil on your chest. Alternatively, you can get relief from congestion and other respiratory problems by boiling eucalyptus leaves in a well-covered pot filled with water then removing the pot's lid to inhale the vapors. This treatment's efficacy is further strengthened by putting a towel over your head and leaning your head over the pot to ensure that you inhale as much vapor as possible. To relieve sore throat, eucalyptus oil can be mixed with warm water to create a mouth rinse. Eucalyptus can help to reduce the duration and intensity of respiratory diseases with its natural antibacterial decongestant properties.

Guaco

This herb significantly promotes a healthy respiratory system. Guaco strengthens the immune system, and it is rich in iron.

Linden

Linden stimulates sweating in order to break a fever. It also helps with flu and cold symptoms such as swollen or inflamed membranes throughout the respiratory tract and the mouth. It also reduces sore throat, irritation, and coughing. In tea form, linden helps to boost the immune system and also eliminates congestion.

Mullein

It is another herb on my list of favorites. It helps to cleanse the lungs and eliminates mucus from the body, especially the lungs. It boosts the circulation of lymph in the neck and chest; it relieves the mucus membrane, and respiratory tract, and also helps to clear congestion. It gives relief for dry cough, asthma, bronchitis, sore throat, and cough.

Sarsaparilla root

This herbal root is highly rich in iron. This makes it essential for the healing of any disease or condition. A patent showed that sarsaparilla possesses therapeutic and preventive agents for allergic and respiratory diseases such as chronic bronchitis, asthmatic bronchitis, bronchial asthma, and acute bronchitis.

Irish Sea Moss

Sea moss contains 92 of the 102 minerals needed for the optimal functioning of the body. These minerals include selenium, potassium, phosphorus, iron, calcium, bromine, iodine, magnesium, and zinc. This herb contains an antiviral property that helps cure respiratory diseases like bronchitis, pneumonia, colds, and flu.

Chapter 15: How to Fast Safely to Remove Mucus, Toxins and Lose Weight by Fasting and its Advantages

What Is Fasting?

The best way to safely fast is the question on the lips of many. Before we delve into that, there is a need to paint a clearer picture of what fasting is. According to Dr. Alvenia Fulton, "The best juices are fresh juices made from your blender out of fresh fruits and vegetables, not from canned or frozen foods."

Before you fast

#1. Fasting comes in two phases in order to cleanse your body effectively. Firstly, you have to cleanse your body with natural herbs for at least five days before embarking on the actual fasting.

   #2. To know when you are ready for fast, your body will give an indication of that, and the indication you are going to get is during the cleansing with herbs phase. When you start feeling hungry while cleansing is when you are truly ready to begin your fast. You should never fast when your body is not ready, if you feel hungry during a fast, you should eat.

Why should you fast?

If you want to know how to correct your body's discomforts, fasting will fix your body and keep you younger. The best method of fasting is to clean the body until there is no more hunger. When there is no hunger, you can fast as long as you like. Fast until your appetite returns because it will disappear. The tongue will become white and soft; fast until the tongue turns red again, and fast until your breath and your body become sweet. The body will produce its own smell due to the removal of all the toxic waste in the body.

What fasting will do

You will look younger, feel younger, skin rejuvenated, and your hair and nails will be revitalized. Fasting will do all these things in your body. If you fast, your body will remain flexible, full of energy, and shine with vitality. This is what we all want, and nothing will do that better than cleansing and fasting. Nothing will do a better job at healing, developing, and relieving our body of waste and toxins if not for fasting (juice, vegetable, or water fasting).

What about Water fasting

Fasting with water is better because it will clean the body of toxic waste, heal the body of old dead cells that have been there for a long time. The best way to do this is to cleanse the body and then start the water fast. When you fast, you will find that your skin becomes resonant, young, and beautiful. Your hair, your eyes, and every gland in your body will respond to fasting. This is what they all need, the intense cleansing that occurs from fasting. If you fast, your friends or people you know can say that you are killing yourself. But I did not listen to them; even during biblical days, people fasted for 21, 30, or 40 days, and no one died of fasting. The prophets, Jesus and the women of the Bible, fasted, and no one died for it. Queen Esther fasted and saved the children of Israel from extinction. Fasting is a way of life.

How to prepare for fasting

Your fasting should start with cleansing. Use different natural herbs for 3 to 5 days before starting your fast, be it a juice, a vegetable, or water fast. Take herbs first to remove some of the toxin and body waste. Most people have toxins that have been in their bodies since they were babies, so herbs are very important before any type of fasting. For example, the first time I tried fasting, on the 21st day, I could not get up quickly enough to go to the bathroom because I had a lot of toxins coming out of me.

How long should you fast?

After cleaning the body with herbs, fast for 21 or 30 days until you no longer have a "coated" tongue, you no longer feel tired, weak, or nervous and feel young again. The people around you will ask you what you are doing; you will look more youthful. Then, break the fast and begin again; if you cleanse the body quickly and adequately, you do not need to take a drug to do what you want. Male or female, your sex drive will continue to work well, and your hormones will work if they are cleansed and quickly.

Fast to cleanse toxins

Our ancestors do not have prostate glands problems like the young men of nowadays. Our grandmothers as well did not lose their youthful factor as it is in today's world. As a matter of fact, my great-grandmother had twin babies at the age of 49, but this is unheard of in the 21st century despite all the medical discoveries. When we eat according to what nature has in store for us, we will stay healthy, live longer, and vanish every pain in the body. Good health will ultimately triumph when we cleanse our bodies and stick to the right diet.

How do you break a fast

You are to break a fast exactly the way you started. By this, I mean, get a juice, warm it up and take that for 5 consecutive days. You will have more energy than you need. You won't feel hungry. If you jump right into taking steaks after an extensive fasting period, you will get sick.

That food will make you fall ill. You have to stop all those kinds of food as they cause body pains and ache. You did not come to this world to live a short life. There are so many ways to fast. The aim of this guide and information therein is to know the correct way for you to fast. In the end, this is all about choosing a fasting method that works well for you.

Advantages of Losing Weight By Dr. Sebi's Fasting Method

Dr. Sebi's Fasting Method Promotes Blood-Sugar Control. By diminishing insulin opposition, which implies your body is progressively viable at moving glucose from your circulation system to your cells, fasting improves glucose control. This advantage is all the more unmistakably found in transient discontinuous fasting; for instance, swearing off nourishment for 18 hours per day, and eating in a six-hour window.

Dr. Sebi's Fasting Method Fights Inflammation. Aggravation is a reaction of devouring an excessive number of acidic-shaping nourishments, poisons, or by being around a lethal situation. Irritation is additionally engaged with the improvement of interminable conditions, for example, coronary illness, disease, numerous sclerosis, and rheumatoid joint pain. By fasting for just 12 hours every day, it is conceivable to diminish irritation, which helps in treating the sicknesses.

Dr. Sebi's Fasting Method Enhances Heart Health. Coronary illness is one of the main sources of death around the globe. By making way of life changes, for example, following Dr. Sebi's Nutritional Guide, and consolidating fasting into your daily practice, it is conceivable to diminish hypertension, triglycerides, and cholesterol, all of which can prompt coronary illness.

Dr. Sebi's Fasting Method Boosts Brain Function. Fasting does beneficial things for the cerebrum, and this is clear by the entirety of the useful neurochemical changes that occur in the mind when we quick. It additionally improves subjective capacity, increments neurotrophic factors and stress opposition, and decreases aggravation. You can help the cerebrum advantages of fasting by devouring Banju while you quick. Dr. Sebi's Banju animates the mind and aids in the treatment of sicknesses identified with the focal sensory system, for example, sorrow, nervousness, peevishness, and a sleeping disorder.

Dr. Sebi's Fasting Method Can Delay Aging and Increase Longevity. Hoping to live more? Take a stab at consolidating fasting strategy as suggested by Dr. Sebi into your daily schedule, as it's demonstrated to postpone maturing and increment life span to the individuals who practice it alongside another solid way of life decisions.

Chapter 16: The 10 Secrets of Dr. Sebi's Diet

Dr. Sebi discovered many things during his lifetime. He also taught a lot of people many things. During his life, he did many interviews and performed at a lot of speaking engagements, where he shared his secrets. Here, we will discuss his top ten diet secrets.

We Have to Go Back to the Mother

Dr. Sebi wrote a paper many years ago called Back to the Mother. In this, he talks about how the land provides for us in a specific manner. He speaks specifically about Africans and how they originally only had the land to live off of. That land provided the foods that they survived with, and that didn't include things like cows, potatoes, beans, yams, lambs, or rice. The lamb came from Arabia and the cow came from Europe. The foods they ate were electric, which is what their body needs and that is what kept them healthy. Today, people have strayed from those ways because now they have access to foods from all over the world. Dr. Sebi explained this by saying that "you don't feed gorillas polar bear food." The problems we have are because we have been given the wrong types of foods. This is the main point of his diet. He wants us to go back to the foods that our bodies want us to eat so that it is able to work properly and to its full capacity.

If you look at how other animals eat, you will notice something very different. Polar bears feed on seals. Hummingbirds feed on the nectar in flowers. Giraffes eat leaves. Among animals, you have herbivores and carnivores. But when it comes to humans, we don't eat the way our people ate centuries ago when food wasn't as prevalent. That means we aren't giving our bodies what it needs because we can't decide if we need meats or need herbs.

Fasting is Key to Healing your Body From Disease

When people hear the word fasting, they instinctively get defensive. When people think fasting, they think starvation, but that isn't what happens when you fast the Dr. Sebi way. Dr. Sebi fasted for 90 days, and it helps to cure his diabetes and impotence. During those 90 days, he learned exactly what it was that people needed in order to heal. During this time, he began to drink his urine, lost his eyesight, but continued to do what he was supposed to do. Then, four days later his eyesight returned.

This was when he started to have everybody fast that was sick, which included his mother. This helped to cure her diabetes and cleared out her excess mucus in 57 days. Fasting does not mean that you give up food altogether. There are actually many different types of fast, and simply eating only the foods in his nutritional guide will put your body into a state of fasting. You can take things a step further by cutting out most foods except for dates when you feel rather weak and drinking bromide plus tea along with plain salads. Fasting is a wonderful thing, and you can experiment with fasting to see what works best for you.

The Body Works Properly through Chemical Affinity

During the trial in the late 80s that Dr. Sebi had to face, he asked the judge if it wasn't true that science had proven the body was carbon-based and that for a carbon-based being to function correctly it needs carbon-based foods. This is what science calls chemical affinity. The body can only accept things that it is made of, not something new or alien to it. The foods that are able to provide you with what your body needs are electric foods. The body likes these foods because it makes its chemical makeup.

There Is only One Disease, and that Is Excess Mucus

While this is quite possibly the most controversial part of Dr. Sebi's teachings, he has repeated time and time that the only disease is too much mucus. When it comes to diseases like diabetes, HIV/AIDS, lupus, and so on, they are created by the body, creating too much mucus in a certain area. The body needs mucus, and it contains several mucous membranes that keep things lubricated. When we eat the wrong foods or do things that cause our bodies to become acidic, mucus starts to grow. The illness that you develop will depend on where all of that mucus begins to grow.

For people with diabetes, the pancreas is where the mucous grows. For something like bronchitis, the mucus is in the lungs. During his trial in the 80s, he asked the judge if she had ever been to an AIDS ward, and she told him yes. Then he asked what the AIDS patients spit up, and she replied with "mucus." That is the basis for his diet is to cleanse the cells of all of this excess mucus to help heal the body from diseases.

Sick People Need Large Doses of Iron Phosphate

When asked by potential patients where they should start, he always tells them to start taking iron, which is found in his Bio Ferra product. Iron phosphates help the cells remain healthy once they have been freed of their excess mucus. Modern medicine tends to give people lots of ferrous oxides. Iron is the only magnetic mineral on the planet. Iron pulls all other minerals to it, so when you take iron, you are also taking all other minerals as well.

The Body is not Designed to Become Sick

The body was not created to become sick. Birds don't get sick. Elephants don't get sick. They don't need a vet. Lions and giraffes don't need a vet, and neither do any of the natural animals. If this is true, then why do humans get sick so often? Why do we suffer from problems like hay fever and allergies? We have violated the laws of nature. We would all probably be happy and okay with this as long as we remain happy until the day we die. But the thing is, we don't stay happy until the day we die. The violation, we have made it has stressed our mind and our body. If you stay in this violation, you will be stressed until the day you die.

So, what is this violation? This violation originated with creation. We forget about creation and the violation occurs when we forget what is said in Genesis.

Carbon, Hydrogen, and Oxygen Are the Main Players in Maintaining Life

This may seem extremely obvious because we are taught this in elementary science classes. Everything that the Universe creates is made up of carbon, hydrogen, and oxygen. Those are the main players in making something organic, and these are often missing from things that are created in a lab. These substances do not have starch in them. All substances that are created by Universe and that are organic will not contain starch.

All of these foods that are naturally present on the Earth, that was made in the Universe, are all alkaline foods. These are all-natural. Our blood and body prefer to be fed by these foods because it does not like starch. Starch is only present because it binds things together. Things only have to be bound together if they are not meant to be together naturally.

You Have to Cleanse and then Rebuild the Body

Dr. Sebi's diet works in two parts. First, when you start following his diet, you will be cleansing your cells, which he called inter-cellular cleansing. This removes toxins and impurities from your body, which will help heal you from any diseases you are suffering from. Once the cells in your body have been cleansed, it will move into the second part, which is rebuilding the body. This means that the body is brought back to its optimal functioning, and most likely to a state that you have never known. The best way for your body to be able to rebuild itself is through the use of iron. If you make sure that your iron level is where it is supposed to be, then you cannot get sick.

Spinach is Not a True Iron-Rich Food Because it is Not Alkaline

As you know already, iron is a very important part of Dr. Sebi's diet. Most everybody will tell you that spinach is a great iron source, but Dr. Sebi will tell you it is not. Spinach is acidic food. It falls below a 6 on the pH scale because it has a starch base. That means it is not natural. The Universe didn't naturally make this, so it is not a good source of iron and will not help your body in any way. On the other hand, moringa has 25 times the amount of iron than spinach does and is not acidic. It also has 14 times the amount of calcium as milk.

The Original Doctor, Hypocrites, didn't Use Chemicals, but Herbs

People have fought the notion of Dr. Sebi's diet for years. To them, it doesn't make sense that people would try to heal themselves with diet and herbs since we have doctors. What they don't realize is that the father of modern medicine, Hypocrites, did things very similar to Dr. Sebi. Back when Hypocrites started practicing medicine, they didn't have the chemicals we have now. He didn't give everybody antibiotics whenever they had the sniffles. They didn't have chemotherapy or radiation. All he had to use were things that grew naturally around him. He wouldn't be considered the father of modern medicine if he hadn't been a successful doctor, yet his practice was very different from todays. So, if you, or anybody you know, want to shake your head at the teachings of Dr. Sebi, just remember that Hypocrites would support what he is doing.

Now you have the ten secrets of Dr. Sebi's diet. While he may have been a completely self-educated man, we knew what he was talking about. Through common sense and personal studies, he created something that has helped many people.

18

Chapter 17: Alkaline Diet Recipes

Trying out some alkaline recipes is a good first step towards a healthier lifestyle. Alkaline diets have long been known to reduce the chance of disease and boost energy. These great benefits are achieved by providing your body with the nutrients it needs to work at its optimum potential. The term "alkaline" in the diet is used to indicate foods that are "alkaline-forming" once metabolized by the body. Different foods are classified as alkaline-forming or acid-forming. By eating a wealth portion of alkaline-forming foods and staying away from acid-forming foods, alkaline diets can help reduce the chances of developing certain diseases.

Examples of such diseases include osteoporosis, inflammation, problems with the urinary tract, digestive problems, and a host of other diseases. Eating alkaline food gives your body the tools it needs to maintain a healthy state. Maintaining an alkaline lifestyle can even help prevent cancer. Check the alkalinity of your body often and keep track of where you are. We know for sure that alkaline-based foods are healthier choices. So the use of these alkaline diet recipes will improve your overall health and lifestyle.

What Is Required Of The Alkaline Diet?

Knowing what to eat may sometimes take some time to figure out when you follow an alkaline diet. An easy thumb rule is to follow the 80/20 rule. When choosing your meals, 80 percent of foods eaten on a diet should be alkaline, while the other 20 percent may be low to medium-acid. Highly acidic food is not recommended.

So how are you going to figure out which foods are alkaline and which are acidic or even highly acidic?

Well, that's the problem most people have when starting an alkaline diet— learn what food to eat!

Making the Transition from Acid to Alkaline

One of the hardest parts of any diet plan is the transition to it. Right now, we've got a specific mind embedded in us. Food companies have spent a lot of money to make us believe that processed food tastes better. In fact, what happened was that our taste buds got used to these foods. Once you start eating whole foods, you'll realize that they actually taste a lot better. But first, we've got to get there, and that's hard!

Simple Tips to Get Started

- Keep things simple. Most people are trying to over comply with their diet. They end up frustrated and angry. There is no need to count calories at first. Just concentrate on filling your plate with alkaline-based food and work from there.
- Drink a lot of water. Hydration is the key to any kind of diet. Most of the people spend most of their mornings dehydrated. Actually, there's a quick fix for this, and it works! Squeeze some lemon juice in a glass of water and drink it. This is the first thing you do every morning. It compensates for the dehydration that you accumulate while sleeping and provides an increase in alkalinity.
- Never deprive yourself of it. It's not working! You've got to remove the food slowly. Don't take all of them away at once. Slowly work towards the 80/20 ratio.
- Don't depend on the power of will alone. Remove all the unsafe food from your home. If you keep unsafe food close to you, you'll eventually be in a cave. There are many yummy alkaline-friendly recipes that you can use

to replace junk food.

- Remove your junk. Remove processed and packaged food slowly.
- Exercise every day. I know this is part of every kind of diet. I've seen a lot of advice given about what the best exercise is. But do you know the best kind of exercise? It's the one you're actually going to do! Just stay active, and you'll be all right.
- Take action now! Knowledge is powerful, but it doesn't matter if you don't take action.

Find out what protocol you can take today and do it. You're responsible for your own health. Make changes that work towards a long-term goal.

Start the Day Off with A Smoothie!

Smoothies serve as a great dietary tool that can be used to detox your body. They're also a wonderful opportunity to put greens in your diet. Plus, they're giving you an alkaline boost so you can get off on the right track.

Energy-enhancing smoothies are our favorite choice because they can replace coffee. Most people don't even know how much energy they are going to waste with their poor choices. Get your fiber.

The "Upbeat" Strawberry and Clementine Glass

Preparation Time: 5 minutes
Cooking Time: 20 minutes
Servings: 2
Ingredients:

- 8 ounces strawberries, fresh
- 1 banana, chopped into chunks
- 2 Clementines/Mandarins

Directions:

1. Peel the Clementines and remove seeds.

2. Add the listed ingredients to your blender/food processor and blend until smooth.
3. Serve chilled and enjoy!

Nutrition:

Calories: 344
Fat: 110.1 g
Carbs: 25.3 g
Protein: 4.8 g
Fiber: 4.9 g

Cabbage and Coconut Chia Smoothie

Preparation Time: 5 minutes
Cooking Time: 20 minutes
Servings: 2
Ingredients:

- 1/3 cup cabbage
- 1 cup cold unsweetened coconut milk
- 1 tablespoon chia seeds
- ½ cup cherries
- ½ cup spinach

Directions:

1. Add coconut milk to your blender.
2. Cut cabbage and add to your blender.
3. Place chia seeds in a coffee grinder and chop to powder, brush the powder into your blender.
4. Pit the cherries and add them to your blender.
5. Wash and dry the spinach and chop.
6. Add to the mix.
7. Cover and blend on low followed by medium. Serve chilled!

Nutrition:

Calories: 274

Fat: 34.1 g

Carbs: 25.3 g

Protein: 4.8 g

Fiber: 4.9 g

The Cherry Beet Delight

Preparation Time: 5 minutes

Cooking Time: 20 minutes

Servings: 2

Ingredients:

- 1 cup cherries, pitted
- ½ cup beets
- Few banana slices
- 1 cup water, filtered, alkaline
- 1 cup coconut milk
- Pinch of organic vanilla powder
- Pinch of cinnamon
- Pinch of stevia
- Few mint leaves/lime slices to garnish

Directions:

1. Add berries, beets, water, banana slices, and coconut milk to your blender. Blend well until smooth. Then add more water if the texture is too creamy for you.
2. Add coconut oil, vanilla, cinnamon, and stir. Add a bit of stevia for extra sweetness.
3. Garnish with mint leaves and lime slices

Nutrition:

Calories: 204

Fat: 10.1 g

Carbs: 25.3 g

Protein: 4.8 g

Fiber: 4.9 g

The Avocado Paradise

Preparation Time: 5 minutes

Cooking Time: 20 minutes

Servings: 2

Ingredients:

- ½ avocado, cubed
- 1 cup coconut milk
- Half a lemon
- ¼ cup fresh spinach leaves
- 1 pear
- 1 tablespoon hemp. Seed powder
- Toppings
- Handful of macadamia nuts
- Handful of grapes
- 2 lemon slices

Directions:

1. Blend all the ingredients until smooth.
2. Add a few ice cubes to make it chilled.
3. Add your desired toppings.

Enjoy!

Nutrition:

Calories: 294

Fat: 310.1 g

Carbs: 25.3 g

Protein: 4.8 g

Fiber: 4.9 g

The Authentic Vegetable Medley

Preparation Time: 5 minutes

Cooking Time: 20 minutes

Servings: 2

Ingredients:

- 1 cup broccoli, steamed
- 1 bunch asparagus, steamed
- 2 cups coconut milk
- 2 tablespoons coconut oil
- 2 carrots, peeled
- Few inch horseradish
- Himalayan salt
- Pinch of chili powder
- ½ an onion
- 2 garlic cloves

Directions:

1. Add all the listed ingredients to your blender except coconut oil, salt and chili powder.
2. Blend until smooth. Add salt, coconut oil, and chili powder.
3. Stir well, and serve chilled!

Nutrition:

Calories: 204

Fat: 10.1 g

Carbs: 25.3 g

Protein: 4.8 g

Fiber: 4.9 g

The Original Power Producer

Preparation Time: 5 minutes

Cooking Time: 20 minutes

Servings: 2

Ingredients:

- ½ cup spinach
- 1 avocado, diced
- 1 cup coconut milk
- 1 tablespoon flax seed
- 2 nori sheets, roasted and crushed
- 1 garlic clove
- Salt to taste
- Toppings
- Handful of pistachios
- 3 tablespoons bell pepper, finely chopped
- A handful of parsley leaves

Directions:

1. Blend all the ingredients until smooth.
2. Add a few ice cubes to make it chilled. Add your desired toppings.

Enjoy!

Nutrition:

Calories: 224

Fat: 560.1 g

Carbs: 25.3 g

Protein: 4.8 g

Fiber: 4.9 g

The Dreamy Cherry Mix

Preparation Time: 5 minutes

Cooking Time: 20 minutes

Servings: 2

Ingredients:

- ½ cup ripe cherries
- Juice of 1 lemon
- 1 cup coconut milk
- 1 avocado, cubed
- ¼ cup spinach
- Few slices of cucumber, peeled
- Toppings
- Handful of pistachios
- Handful of raisins
- 1 slice lemon

Directions:

1. Blend all the ingredients until smooth.
2. Add a few ice cubes to make it chilled.
3. Add your desired toppings.

Enjoy!

Nutrition:

Calories: 232

Fat: 21.1 g

Carbs: 25.3 g

Protein: 4.8 g

Fiber: 4.9 g

Better than Your Favorite Restaurant "Lemon Smoothie"

Preparation Time: 5 minutes
Cooking Time: 20 minutes
Servings: 2
Ingredients:

· 2 cups organic rice milk, gluten free
· 1 cup melon, chopped
· ½ an avocado, cubed
· ½ a cucumber, peeled and sliced
· Ice cubes
· 2 limes, juiced
· 1 tablespoon coconut oil
· Few banana slices to taste

Directions:

1. Add the listed ingredients to your blender (except coconut oil) and blend well.
2. Blend until you have a smooth texture.
3. Add coconut oil and stir.

Enjoy!

Nutrition:
Calories: 204
Fat: 10.1 g
Carbs: 25.3 g
Protein 4.8 g
Fiber 4.9 g

The "One" With the Watermelon
Preparation Time: 5 minutes

Cooking Time: 20 minutes
Servings: 2
Ingredients:

- 1 cup watermelon, sliced
- ½ cup coconut, shredded
- 1 grapefruit, cubed
- ½ cup coconut milk
- 2 tablespoons almond butter
- Toppings
- Handful of crushed almonds
- Handful of raisins
- 2 tablespoons coconut powder

Directions:

1. Blend all the ingredients until smooth
2. Add a few ice cubes to make it chilled
3. Add your desired toppings

Enjoy!

Nutrition:

Calories 284
Fat: 10.1 g
Carbs: 25.3 g
Protein: 14.8 g
Fiber: 564.9 g

The Sweet Potato Acid Buster

Preparation Time: 5 minutes
Cooking Time: 20 minutes
Servings: 2

Ingredients:

- 1 cup sweet potato, chopped
- 1 cup almond milk
- ¼ teaspoon nutmeg
- ¼ teaspoon ground cinnamon
- 1 teaspoon flax seed
- 1 small avocado, cubed
- Few spinach leaves, torn
- Toppings
- Handful of crushed almonds
- Handful of crushed cashews
- 3 tablespoons orange juice

Directions:

1. Blend all the ingredients until smooth.
2. Add a few ice cubes to make it chilled. Add your desired toppings.

Enjoy!

Nutrition:

Calories: 784

Fat: 10.1 g

Carbs: 25.3 g

Protein: 14.8 g

Fiber: 564.9 g

Matcha Coconut Smoothie

Preparation Time: 5 minutes

Cooking Time: 20 minutes

Servings: 2

Ingredients:

- 1 whole banana, cubed
- 1 cup frozen mango, chunked
- 2 kale leaves, torn
- 3 tablespoon white beans
- 2 tablespoon shredded coconut
- ½ teaspoon matcha green tea powder
- 1 cup water

Directions:

1. Add banana, kale, mango, matcha powder and white beans to your blender.
2. Blend until you have a nice smoothie.
3. Add shredded coconut as topping.
4. Serve and enjoy!

Nutrition:

Calories 249
Fat: 10.1 g
Carbs: 25.3 g
Protein: 14.8 g
Fiber 564.9 g

19

Chapter 18: Dr. Sebi's Approved Recipes

Welcome to another way of eating and healthful living. Think of it as an excursion. It isn't always easy to quit eating the many acidic foods we've enjoyed for such a long time and have gotten addicted to - but surely, we can accomplish the best diet through cleansing and supporting our bodies with the foods the Creator has given. These plans convey the years of healing and sharing testimonies by our customers, companions, and staff.

Dr. Sebi's Organic Foods

For optimal health, we must eat just non-hybridized organically developed produce. Chemical producers develop conventional or industrial products with pesticides, herbicides, manufactured manures, and different chemicals that are poisonous and harmful to the body. Food producers develop organic foods without using these toxic substances; in this way, they are nutritious, taste better, and are less dangerous to our bodies.

Raw Vs. Cooked

During the vast majority of our reality on this planet, what decisions do we have for food? What have we been eating during the initial 50,000 years before we found fire, tools, and murder animals for consumptions? The original diet of Homo sapiens more likely to have been vegetables, fruits, and nuts!

Eating Properly

Are you addicted to food? Many of us have gotten addicted to certain foods. Nature addicts many people to about 5 or 6 foods, and these foods are inconvenient for them to abstain from eating. These foods are usually crossbreeding and incorporate rice, beans, soy, bread, potatoes, potato chips, espresso, teas, desserts, chocolate candy, fish, and carrot juice. Because of the high substance of sugar, cigarettes are another addiction for many.

Strawberry and Chia Seed Overnight Oats Parfait

Preparation Time: 5 minutes

Cooking Time: 5 minutes

Servings: 2

Ingredients:

For the Strawberry Mixture

- 1 cup diced strawberries.
- 1 teaspoon chia seeds.
- 1 to 2 teaspoons brown rice syrup.

For the Oat Mixture

- 1 cup quick rolled oats.
- 1 cup coconut milk (boxed).
- 1 tablespoon brown rice syrup.
- ⅛ tablespoon vanilla bean powder.

Directions:

1. In a small bowl, stir together the strawberries, chia seeds, and brown rice syrup until well combined.
2. In a small bowl, stir together the oats, coconut milk, brown rice syrup,

and vanilla bean powder until well combined.

3. Place half the oat mixture in the bottom of 1 large glass mason jar or 2 small jars, and layer half of the strawberry mixture over the oat mixture. Repeat with the remaining oat and strawberry mixtures.

4. Cover the mason jar(s), and refrigerate overnight.

5. Uncover and enjoy.

Nutrition:

Calories: 192

Fat: 8 g

Carbs: 31.3 g

Protein: 4.2 g

Fiber: 5.4 g

Carrot and Hemp Seed Muffins

Preparation Time: 5 minutes

Cooking Time: 5 minutes

Servings: 2

Ingredients:

- 3 tablespoons water
- 1 tablespoon ground flaxseed
- 2 cups oat flour
- 1 cup almond milk (boxed)
- ½ cup unrefined whole cane sugar, such as Sucanat
- 1 carrot, shredded
- 6 tablespoons cashew butter
- 2 tablespoons hemp seeds
- 1 tablespoon chopped lacinato kale
- 1 tablespoon baking powder
- ⅛ teaspoon vanilla bean powder
- Pinch sea salt

Directions:

1. Preheat the oven to 350°F.
2. To prepare a flax egg, in a small bowl, whisk together the water and flaxseed.
3. Transfer the flax egg to a medium bowl, and add the oat flour, almond milk, sugar, carrot, cashew butter, hemp seeds, kale, baking powder, vanilla bean powder, and salt, stirring until well combined.
4. Divide the mixture evenly among 12 muffin cups, bake for 20 to 25 minutes, and enjoy right away.

Nutrition:

Calories: 292

Fat: 8 g

Carbs: 31.3 g

Protein: 4.2 g

Fiber: 5.4

Raspberry-Avocado Smoothie Bowl

Preparation Time: 5 minutes

Cooking Time: 0 minutes

Servings: 2

Ingredients:

- 1½ cups coconut milk (boxed)
- 1 cup raspberries, plus more (optional) for topping
- 1 avocado, roughly chopped
- 3 tablespoons unrefined whole cane sugar, such as Sucanat, divided
- 1 teaspoon chia seeds
- 1 teaspoon unsweetened shredded coconut
- Mixed berries, for topping (optional)

Directions:

1. In a blender, blend to combine the coconut milk, raspberries, avocado, and 2 tablespoons of sugar until smooth and creamy.
2. Pour the mixture into 2 serving bowls, sprinkle the extra raspberries (if using), the remaining 1 tablespoon of the sugar, and the chia seeds, shredded coconut, and mixed berries (if using) over the top, and enjoy.

Nutrition:
Calories: 102
Fat: 8 g
Carbs: 31.3 g
Protein 4.2 g
Fiber 5.4 g

Sweet Potato and Kale Breakfast Hash
Preparation Time: 15 minutes
Cooking Time: 15 minutes
Servings: 2
Ingredients:

- 1 teaspoon avocado oil
- 2 cups peeled and cubed sweet potatoes
- ½ cup chopped kale
- ½ cup diced onion
- ½ teaspoon sea salt
- ½ teaspoon freshly ground black pepper
- ½ avocado, cubed (optional)
- 1 to 2 teaspoons sesame seeds or hemp seeds (optional)

Directions:

1. In a large skillet over medium heat, heat the avocado oil. Add the sweet potatoes, kale, onion, salt, and pepper, and sauté for 10 to 15 minutes, or until the sweet potatoes are soft. Remove from the heat.

2. Gently stir in the avocado and sesame seeds (if using), transfer to 1 large or 2 small plates, and enjoy.

Nutrition:

Calories: 202

Fat: 6 g

Carbs: 31.3 g

Protein: 4.2 g

Fiber: 5.4 g

Avocados with Kale and Almond Stuffing

Preparation Time: 5 minutes

Cooking Time: 0 minutes

Servings: 2

Ingredients:

- ½ cup almonds
- ½ cup chopped lacinato kale
- 1 garlic clove
- ½ jalapeño
- 2 tablespoons nutritional yeast
- 1 tablespoon avocado oil
- 1 tablespoon apple cider vinegar
- 1 tablespoon freshly squeezed lemon juice
- ¼ teaspoon sea salt
- 1 avocado, halved and pitted

Directions:

1. In a food processor, pulse the almonds, kale, garlic, jalapeño, nutritional yeast, avocado oil, apple cider vinegar, lemon juice, and sea salt until everything is well combined, the almonds are in small pieces, and it has a chunky texture, taking care not to over process.

2. Add half of the stuffing mixture to the center of each avocado half, and enjoy.

Nutrition:
Calories: 192
Fat: 8 g
Carbs: 31.3 g
Protein: 4.2 g
Fiber: 5.4 g

Mixed Berry–Chia Seed Pudding
Preparation Time: 5 minutes
Cooking Time: 5 minutes
Servings: 2
Ingredients:

- 1 cup coconut milk (boxed)
- ½ cup mixed berries (raspberries, blackberries, blueberries), plus more (optional) for topping
- 2 tablespoons chia seeds
- 1 to 2 tablespoons unrefined whole cane sugar, such as Sucanat

Directions:

1. In a mason jar, combine the coconut milk, berries, chia seeds, and sugar, adjusting the sugar to your preference.
2. Seal the jar tightly, and shake vigorously until well mixed.
3. Refrigerate for about 1 hour, or until the pudding thickens to your preference.
4. Stir, top with the extra mixed berries (if using), and enjoy.

Nutrition:
Calories: 122

Fat: 18 g

Carbs: 31.3 g

Protein: 114.2 g

Fiber: 5.4 g

Pineapple and Coconut Oatmeal Bowl

Preparation Time: 5 minutes

Cooking Time: 5 minutes

Servings: 2

Ingredients:

For The Oatmeal

- 1 cup quick rolled oats
- 1 (13.5-ounce) can full-fat coconut milk
- 2 tablespoons unrefined whole cane sugar, such as Sucanat

For Assembling

- ½ cup cubed pineapple
- ¼ cup unsweetened coconut flakes
- 1 tablespoon chia seeds
- 1 tablespoon pumpkin seeds, chopped

Directions:

1.In a small saucepan over medium-low heat, cook the oats, coconut milk, and sugar for 3 to 5 minutes or until the oats are soft; adjust the sugar to your preference.

To Assemble

2.Transfer the oatmeal to 2 serving bowls, top with the cubed pineapple, coconut flakes, and chia and pumpkin seeds, and serve.

Nutrition:

Calories: 371

Fat: 12.5 g

Carbs: 31.3 g

Protein: 4.2 g

Fiber: 5.4 g

Vanilla Bean and Cinnamon Granola

Preparation Time: 5 minutes

Cooking Time: 5 minutes

Servings: 2

Ingredients:

- 3 cups quick rolled oats
- ½ cup brown rice syrup
- 6 tablespoons coconut oil
- ¼ cup unrefined whole cane sugar, such as Sucanat
- 2 teaspoons vanilla bean powder
- 2 teaspoons ground cinnamon
- ¼ teaspoon sea salt

Directions:

1. Preheat the oven to 250°F. Line a baking pan with parchment paper.
2. In a large bowl, use your hands to mix together the oats, brown rice syrup, coconut oil, sugar, vanilla bean powder, cinnamon, and salt until well combined.
3. Squeeze the mixture together into a ball, and transfer to the prepared baking pan.
4. Press the mixture evenly on the baking pan, taking care not to break it up into small pieces. This will allow it to bake in large cluster pieces that you can break apart after baking, if you prefer.
5. Bake for about 30 minutes, or until crispy, taking care not to overbake.

6. Cool completely before serving. The granola will harden and get even crispier as it cools. Store in an airtight container.

Nutrition:

Calories: 341

Fat: 11.8 g

Carbs: 31.3 g

Protein 412.2 g

Fiber 5.4 g

Sesame and Hemp Seed Breakfast Cookies

Preparation Time: 5 minutes

Cooking Time: 5 minutes

Servings: 2

Ingredients:

- ⅔ cup cashew butter
- ½ cup quick rolled oats
- ¼ cup hemp seeds
- ¼ cup sesame seeds
- 3 tablespoons brown rice syrup
- 3 tablespoons coconut oil, melted
- 1 teaspoon vanilla bean powder
- 1 teaspoon ground cinnamon

Directions:

1. Line a baking sheet with parchment paper.
2. In a medium bowl, stir together the cashew butter, oats, hemp seeds, sesame seeds, brown rice syrup, coconut oil, vanilla bean powder, and cinnamon until well combined.
3. Refrigerate the bowl for 5 to 10 minutes to allow the mixture to firm up.

4. Scoop a tablespoonful of dough at a time and flatten it into a disk with your hands. Smooth the outer edges with your fingertips, and place them on the prepared baking sheet. Repeat with the remaining dough.

5. Refrigerate the cookies for about 20 minutes or until they firm up, and serve. Store leftovers in an airtight container in the refrigerator; they will soften and lose their shape at room temperature.

Nutrition:

Calories: 119

Fat: 28.7 g

Carbs: 31.3 g

Protein: 74.2 g

Fiber: 5.4 g

Fresh Fruit with Vanilla-Cashew Cream

Preparation Time: 5 minutes

Cooking Time: 5 minutes

Servings: 4

Ingredients:

- Room-temperature water, for soaking
- 1 cup raw cashews
- 1 (13.5-ounce) can coconut milk
- 2 tablespoons brown rice syrup
- 2 tablespoons unrefined whole cane sugar, such as Sucanat
- 2 teaspoons vanilla bean powder
- 1 teaspoon freshly squeezed lemon juice
- ¼ teaspoon ground cinnamon
- ¼ teaspoon sea salt

Directions:

1. 4 cups alkaline fruit, such as raspberries, blackberries, blueberries, strawberries, mango, pineapple, or cantaloupe
2. In a medium bowl with enough room-temperature water to cover them, soak the cashews for 15 to 20 minutes.
3. Drain and rinse the cashews.
4. In a high-speed blender, blend to combine the soaked cashews, coconut milk, brown rice syrup, sugar, vanilla bean powder, lemon juice, cinnamon, and salt until creamy and smooth. Add more sugar, if you like.
5. Add 1 cup of fruit to each of 4 serving bowls, drizzle each bowl of fruit with ½ cup of cream, and serve.

Nutrition:

Calories: 412
Fat: 28.1g
Carbs: 31.9g
Protein: 41.2g
Fiber: 15.4g

20

Chapter 19: Salad Recipes

Mango & Avocado Salad

Preparation Time: 15 minutes

Cooking Time: 0 minutes

Servings: 6

Ingredients:

- 2½ cups mango, peeled, pitted and sliced
- 2½ cups avocado, peeled, pitted and sliced
- 1 red onion, sliced
- 6 cups fresh baby arugula
- ¼ cup fresh mint leaves, chopped
- 2 tablespoons fresh orange juice
- Sea salt, as required

Directions:

1. Place all the ingredients in a large serving bowl and gently, toss to combine.
2. Cover and refrigerate to chill before serving.

Nutrition:

Calories: 182

Fat: 12.3g

Carbs: 18.8g

Protein: 2.6g

Fiber: 6.2g

Cucumber & Tomato Salad

Preparation Time: 15 minutes

Cooking Time: 0 minutes

Servings: 6

Ingredients:

- 2 cups plum tomatoes, chopped
- 2 cups cucumbers, chopped
- 3 cups Bibb lettuce, torn
- 3 cups fresh baby kale
- 2 tablespoons olive oil
- 2 tablespoons fresh key lime juice
- Sea salt, as required

Directions:

1. In a large serving bowl, place all the ingredients and gently, toss to combine.
2. Serve immediately.

Nutrition:

Calories: 80

Fat: 4.9g

Carbs: 8.7g

Protein: 2.1g

Fiber: 1.5g

Tomato & Greens Salad

Preparation Time: 15 minutes

Cooking Time: 0 minutes

Servings: 4

Ingredients:

- 6 cups fresh baby arugula
- 2 cups cherry tomatoes
- 2 scallions, chopped
- 2 tablespoons olive oil
- 2 tablespoons fresh orange juice
- Sea salt, as required

Directions:

1. In a large bowl, place all the ingredients and toss to coat well.
2. Cover the bowl and refrigerate for about 6-8 hours.
3. Remove from the refrigerator and toss well before serving.

Nutritions:

Calories: 90

Fat: 7.4g

Carbs: 6g

Protein: 1.8g

Fiber: 1.8g

Mashed Chickpeas Salad

Preparation time: 15 minutes

Cooking Time: 0 minutes

Servings: 4

Ingredients:

For Hemp Seed Mayo

- 1 cup hemp seeds
- ¾ cup spring water
- 2 tbsp. grapeseed oil
- 1 tbsp. onion powder
- 1 tsp. fresh key lime juice
- Sea salt, as required

For Salad

- 2½ cups cooked chickpeas
- ¼ cup red onions, chopped
- ¼ cup green bell peppers, seeded and chopped
- ½ of Nori sheet, cut into small pieces
- 1 teaspoon onion powder
- 1 teaspoon dill
- Sea salt, as required

Directions:

1. For mayo: in a blender, add all the ingredients and pulse on high speed until smooth.
2. For salad: in a bowl, add the chickpeas and with a potato masher, mash until desired texture is reached.
3. Add the remaining ingredients and mix until well combined.
4. Refrigerate to chill for about 40-60 minutes before serving.

Nutrition:
Calories: 403
Fat: 22g
Carbs: 31.1g
Protein: 19.3g
Fiber: 7.6g

Chickpeas & Quinoa Salad

Preparation Time: 20 minutes

Cooking Time: 20 minutes

Servings: 8

Ingredients:

1¾ cups spring water

- 1 cup quinoa, rinsed
- Sea salt, as required
- 2 cups cooked chickpeas
- 1 medium green bell pepper, seeded and chopped
- 1 medium red bell pepper, seeded and chopped
- 2 large cucumbers, chopped
- ½ cup scallion (green part), chopped
- 2 tablespoons olive oil
- 2 tablespoons fresh basil leaves, chopped

Directions:

1. In a pan, add the water over high heat and bring to a boil.
2. Add the quinoa and salt and cook until boiling.
3. Reduce the heat to low and simmer, covered for about 15-20 minutes or until all the liquid is absorbed.
4. Remove from the heat and set aside, covered for about 5-10 minutes.
5. Uncover and with a fork, fluff the quinoa.
6. In a large serving bowl, place the quinoa with the remaining ingredients and gently, toss to coat.
7. Serve immediately.

Nutrition:

Calories: 313

Fat: 5.5g

Carbs: 29.6g

Protein: 7.4g

Fiber: 4.9g

Kale & Orange Salad

Preparation Time: 15 minutes

Cooking Time: 0 minutes

Servings: 2

Ingredients:

For Salad

- 3 cups fresh kale, tough ribs removed and torn
- 2 oranges, peeled and segmented
- 2 tablespoons fresh cranberries
- ¼ teaspoon white sesame seeds

For Dressing

- 2 tablespoons olive oil
- 2 tablespoons fresh orange juice
- ½ teaspoon agave nectar
- Sea salt, as required

Directions:

1. For salad: place all ingredients in a large serving bowl and mix.
2. For dressing: place all ingredients in n another bowl and beat until well combined.
3. Pour the dressing over salad and toss to coat well.
4. Serve immediately.

Nutrition:

Calories: 274

Fat: 14.4g

Carbs: 35.8g

Protein: 4.9g

Fiber: 6.3g

21

Chapter 20: Vegetable Recipe

Sautéed Kale

Preparation Time: 5 minutes

Cooking Time: 4 minutes

Servings: 4

Ingredients:

- 2 tablespoons extra virgin olive oil
- 1 onion, chopped
- 1 large bunch kale, washed and chopped
- 1/2 cup spring water
- A pinch of salt to taste

Directions:

1. Press the Sauté button on the Instant Pot and heat the oil.
2. Sauté the onion for 30 seconds.
3. Stir in the kale and he rest of the ingredients.
4. Close the lid and set the vent to the Sealing position.
5. Press the Manual button and adjust the cooking time to 3 minutes.
6. Do quick pressure release.

Nutrition:

Calories: 46

Fat: 3.2g

Carbs: 4g

Protein: 1.1g

Fiber: 0g

Dr. Sebi's Vegan Ribs

Preparation Time: 5 minutes

Cooking Time: 10 minutes

Servings: 1

Ingredients:

- 2 portobello mushrooms
- 1/2 cup spring water
- 1 teaspoon salt
- 1 teaspoon onion powders
- 1/2 teaspoon cayenne pepper powder
- 1 tablespoon extra-virgin olive oil

Directions:

1. Place all ingredients in the Instant Pot and give a good stir.
2. Close the lid and set the vent to the Sealing position.
3. Press the Manual button and adjust the cooking time to 5 minutes.
4. Once the timer sets off, do quick pressure release.
5. Once the lid is open, press the Sauté button and cook for 5 more minutes until the sauce reduces or thickens.

Nutrition:

Calories: 142

Fat: 7.5g

Carbs: 14.8g

Protein: 8.7g

Fiber: 0g

Sautéed Callaloo

Preparation Time: 3 minutes

Cooking Time: 3 minutes

Servings: 4

Ingredients:

- 1/2 teaspoon coconut oil
- 1 medium onion
- 1 fresh plum tomato, chopped
- A bunch of Callaloo kale or green amaranth
- 1/2 teaspoon oregano
- A sprig of thyme
- A dash of sea salt
- 1/2 cup spring water

Directions:

1. Press the Sauté button on the Instant Pot and heat the oil.
2. Sauté the onion for 30 seconds.
3. Stir in the tomatoes and cook for another 30 seconds.
4. Stir in the kale and season with oregano, thyme, and salt. Pour in water.
5. Close the lid and set the vent to the Sealing position.
6. Press the Manual button and adjust the cooking time to 3 minutes.

Nutrition:

Calories: 29

Fat: 0.8g

Carbs: 5.8g

Protein: 0.6g

Fiber: 0g

Garbanzos with Hemp Nacho Sauce

Preparation Time: 5 minutes

Cooking Time: 20 minutes

Servings: 4

Ingredients:

- 1 cup garbanzos beans, soaked overnight
- 1 cup spring water
- 1 cup shelled hemp seeds
- 1/3 cup spring water
- 1 red bell pepper, seeded and chopped
- 2 tablespoons lemon juice
- 2 tablespoons granulated seaweed
- 1 tablespoon chili powder
- 1/2 teaspoon sea salt

Directions:

1. Place the garbanzos beans and water in the Instant Pot.
2. Close the lid and set the vent to the Sealing position. Press the Steam button and adjust the cooking
3. time to 20 minutes.
4. Do quick pressure release.
5. Once the lid is open, take the garbanzos out and place in a bowl to cool.
6. While the garbanzos are cooling down, place the remaining ingredients in a blender. Pulse until a
7. smooth mixture is formed.
8. Pour the sauce over the broccoli.

Nutrition:

Calories: 405

Fat: 21.4g

Carbs: 41.1g

Protein: 17.9g

Fiber: 0g

Chickpea Tofu

Preparation Time: 3 minutes

Cooking Time: 10 minutes

Servings per Recipe: 4

Ingredients:

- 2 cups spring water
- 1 cup chickpea flour
- 1 teaspoon sea salt

Directions:

1. In a bowl, combine the spring water, chickpea flour, and sea salt. Stir to combine everything.
2. Press the Sauté button on the Instant Pot and pour in the mixture.
3. Constantly mix until the batter thickens. This will take about 10 minutes.
4. Turn off the Instant Pot and pour the thickened batter in a mold.
5. Allow to cool before slicing into cubes.

Nutrition:

Calories: 89

Fat: 1.5g

Carbs: 13.3g

Protein: 5.2g

Fiber: 0g

Simple Dr. Sebi-Approved Vegetarian Stir-Fry

Preparation Time: 3 minutes

Cooking Time: 5 minutes

Servings: 2

Ingredients:

- 1 tablespoon extra-virgin olive oil
- 1 onion, chopped
- 1/2 cup chopped chayote
- 1/2 cup nopales leaves, chopped
- 1/2 cup mushrooms, chopped
- 1/4 teaspoon sea salt
- 1/2 teaspoon spring water

Directions:

1. Press the Sauté button on the Instant Pot.
2. Heat the olive oil and sauté the onion for 30 seconds.
3. Stir in the chayote, nopales leaves, and mushrooms. Season with salt.
4. Add in the spring water.
5. Close the lid and set the vent to the Sealing position.
6. Press the Manual button and adjust the cooking time for 3 minutes.

Nutrition:

Calories: 64

Fat: 3.2g

Carbs: 8.1g

Protein: 1.9g

Fiber: 0g

Garbanzos and Vegetables

Preparation Time: 5 minutes

Cooking Time: 23 minutes
Servings: 4
Ingredients:

- 2 small onions, chopped
- 1 cup garbanzos beans, soaked overnight in water, and rinsed
- 1 cup plum tomatoes, chopped
- 3 cups spring water
- 1/2 teaspoon sea salt
- 1 cup mushrooms, chopped
- 1 cup amaranth greens, chopped

Directions:

1. Place the onions, garbanzos, tomatoes, water, and salt in the Instant Pot. Stir in the mushrooms.
2. Close the lid and seal the vent.
3. Press the Bean/Chili button and cook using the preset cooking time.
4. Once the timer sets off, do quick pressure release.
5. Once the lid is open, press the Sauté button and stir in the amaranth beans.
6. Cook for another 3 minutes until the greens are cooked.

Nutrition:
Calories: 267
Fat: 3.2g
Carbs: 50.8g
Protein: 11.8g
Fiber: 0g

Instant Pot Dr. Sebi-Approved Falafel
Preparation Time: 5 minutes
Cooking Time: 26 minutes

Servings: 4

Ingredients:

- 1 cup raw chickpeas, soaked overnight, and rinsed
- 2 cups spring water
- 1/4 teaspoon sea salt
- 1 tablespoon lemon juice
- 1/2 teaspoon cayenne pepper
- 1/2 teaspoon basil, chopped
- 1/2 teaspoon dill, chopped
- 1/2 cup spelt flour
- Grapeseed oil for frying

Directions:

1. Place the chickpeas and spring water in the Instant Pot. Add salt.
2. Close the lid and press the Bean/Chili button. Cook on high using the pre-set cooking time.
3. Once the timer sets off, do natural pressure release. Drain the chickpeas and allow to cool in a bowl.
4. Once the chickpeas are cool, mash using a fork and add in the lemon juice, cayenne pepper, basil, dill, and spelt flour. Add more sea salt if needed.
5. Mix until everything is well-combined.
6. Using your hands, form small balls using the mixture and set them aside.
7. Into a clean Instant Pot, pour in the grapeseed oil and press the Sauté button until the oil is hot.
8. Fry the falafel balls for 3 minutes on all sides.
9. Serve immediately.

Nutrition:

Calories: 295

Fat: 7g

Carbs: 47.3g

Protein: 13.5g

Fiber: 0g

Vegetable Alfredo

Preparation Time: 5 minutes

Cooking Time: 12 minutes

Servings: 4

Ingredients:

- 1 cup Brazil nuts
- 1/3 cup spring water
- 1 tablespoon granulated seaweed
- 1/2 teaspoon sea salt
- 2 tablespoons lemon juice
- 1 red bell pepper, seeded and chopped
- 1 tablespoon extra-virgin olive oil
- 1 onion, chopped
- 1 orange bell pepper, seeded and chopped
- 10-ounce spelt tortiglioni pasta
- 1 summer squash, seeded and chopped
- 1 cup spring water
- 1/2 cup basil leaves

Directions:

1. Place the Brazil nuts, 1/3 cup spring water, seaweed, sea salt, lemon juice, and red bell pepper in a blender. Pulse until smooth. Set aside.
2. Place the olive oil in the Instant Pot and press the Sauté button. Sauté the onions and bell pepper for 30 seconds.

3. Add in the pasta, summer squash, and water. Season with more salt if desired.
4. Close the lid and set the vent to the Sealing position.
5. Press the Multigrain button and adjust the cooking time to 6 minutes.
6. Do quick pressure release.
7. Once the lid is open, press the Sauté button and pour in the Brazil Nut cheese sauce. Stir and cook for 5 more minutes.
8. Garnish with basil leaves before serving.

Nutrition:
Calories: 499
Fat: 25.7g
Carbs: 60.1g
Protein: 16.1g
Fiber: 0g

Veggies Fajitas
Preparation Time: 3 minutes
Cooking Time: 7 minutes
Servings: 4
Ingredients:

- 1 tablespoon extra-virgin olive oil
- 1-1/2 cup sliced green and red bell peppers, seeded, and chopped
- 1-1/2 cups sliced red onions
- 3 cups sliced mushrooms
- 2 teaspoon sea salt
- 1 tablespoon powdered seaweed
- 1/2 teaspoon cayenne pepper powder
- Juice from 1/2 lime
- 1/2 cup water

Directions:

1. Press the Sauté button on the Instant Pot and heat the olive oil.
2. Sauté the bell peppers and onions for 1 minute until the vegetables have slightly wilted.
3. Stir in the rest of the ingredients.
4. Close the lid and set the vent to the Sealing position.
5. Press the Manual button and adjust the cooking time to 6 minutes.

Nutrition:

Calories: 41
Fat: 1.6g
Carbs: 6.7g
Protein: 1.2g
Fiber: 0g

Baked Garbanzos Beans

Preparation Time: 5 minutes
Cooking Time: 30 minutes
Servings: 4
Ingredients:

- 3 cups garbanzos beans, soaked overnight and rinsed
- 5 cups spring water
- 6 plum tomatoes, chopped
- 3 tablespoons agave
- 1/2 cup date sugar
- 1/4 cup white onions
- 1/4 cup green peppers, seeded and chopped
- 2 teaspoon sea salt
- 1/8 teaspoon cloves
- 1/8 teaspoon cayenne pepper

Directions:

1. To the Instant Pot, place the garbanzos beans and spring water. Close the lid and set the vent to the Sealing position. Press the Bean/Chili button and cook for 20 minutes on high.
2. Meanwhile, place the tomatoes, agave, date sugar, onions, green pepper, salt, cloves, and cayenne pepper in a blender. Pulse until smooth.
3. Once the timer on the Instant Pot sets off, do natural pressure release to open the lid.
4. Drain half of the liquid and pour in the sauce.
5. Close the lid again and set the vent to the Sealing position. Press the Bean/Chili button and cook for another 10 minutes.

Nutrition:
Calories: 692
Fat: 9.7g
Carbs: 125.4g
Protein: 31.2g
Fiber: 0g

Quinoa Taco Meat
Preparation Time: 3 minutes
Cooking Time: 20 minutes
Servings: 2
Ingredients:

- 1 cup red quinoa
- 1-3/4 cup water
- 1/2 teaspoon sea salt
- 1/2 cup plum tomatoes, chopped
- 1 tablespoon powdered seaweed
- 2 teaspoons cayenne pepper powder

- 1/4 cup red onion, chopped

Directions:

1. Place the red quinoa, water, and sea salt in the Instant Pot. Close the lid and set the vent to the Sealing position. Press the Multigrain button and cook on high using the preset cooking time.
2. Once the timer sets off, do natural pressures release. Fluff the quinoa and place in a bowl to cool. Once cool, place the tomatoes, seaweed, cayenned pepper, and red onion into the quinoa. Toss to coat everything.

Nutrition:
Calories: 392
Fat: 5.4g
Carbs: 74.5g
Protein: 13.3g
Fiber: 0g

22

Chapter 21: Snack and Dessert Recipe

Pumpkin Spice Crackers
Preparation Time: 10 minutes
Cooking Time: 1 hour
Servings: 6
Ingredients:

- ⅓ cup coconut flour
- 2 tablespoons pumpkin pie spice
- ¾ cup sunflower seeds
- ¾ cup flaxseed
- ⅓ cup sesame seeds
- 1 tablespoon ground psyllium husk powder
- 1 teaspoon sea salt
- 3 tablespoons coconut oil, melted
- 1⅓ cups alkaline water

Directions:

1. Set your oven to 300 degrees F. Combine all dry ingredients in a bowl.
2. Add water and oil to the mixture and mix well.
3. Let the dough stay for 2 to 3 minutes

4. Spread the dough on a cookie sheet lined with parchment paper.
5. Bake for 30 minutes.
6. Reduce the oven heat to low and bake for another 30 minutes.
7. Crack the bread into bite-size pieces. Serve

Nutrition:

Calories: 248

Fat: 15.7g

Carbs: 0.4g

Protein: 24.9g

Fiber: 0g

Spicy Roasted Nuts

Preparation Time: 10 minutes

Cooking Time: 15 minutes

Servings: 4

Ingredients:

- 8 oz. pecans or coconuts or walnuts
- 1 teaspoon sea salt
- 1 tablespoon olive oil or coconut oil
- 1 teaspoon ground cumin
- 1 teaspoon paprika powder or chili powder

Directions:

1. Add all the ingredients to a skillet.
2. Roast the nuts until golden brown.
3. Serve and enjoy.

Nutrition:

Calories: 287

Fat: 29.5g

Carbs: 5.9g

Protein: 4.2g

Fiber: 4.3g

Wheat Crackers

Preparation Time: 10 minutes

Cooking Time: 20 minutes

Servings: 4

Ingredients:

- 1 3/4 cups coconut flour
- 1 1/2 cups coconut flour
- 3/4 teaspoon sea salt
- 1/3 cup vegetable oil
- 1 cup alkaline water
- Sea salt for sprinkling

Directions:

1. Set your oven to 350 degrees F.
2. Mix coconut flour, coconut flour, and salt in a bowl.
3. Stir in vegetable oil and water. Mix well until smooth.
4. Spread this dough on a floured surface into a thin sheet. Cut small squares out of this sheet.
5. Arrange the dough squares on a baking sheet lined with parchment paper. Bake for 20 minutes until light golden in color.
6. Serve.

Nutrition:

Calories: 64

Fat: 9.2g

Carbs: 9.2g

Protein: 1.5g

Fiber: 0.9g

Potato Chips

Preparation Time: 10 minutes

Cooking Time: 5 minutes

Servings: 4

Ingredients:

- 1 tablespoon vegetable oil
- 1 potato, sliced paper-thin
- Sea salt, to taste

Directions:

1. Toss potato with oil and sea salt.
2. Spread the slices in a baking dish in a single layer.
3. Cook in a microwave for 5 minutes until golden brown.
4. Serve.

Nutrition:

Calories: 80

Fat: 3.5g

Carbs: 11.6g

Protein: 1.2g

Fiber: 0.7g

Zucchini Pepper Chips

Preparation Time: 10 minutes

Cooking Time: 15 minutes

Servings: 4

Ingredients:

- 1 2/3 cups vegetable oil
- 1 teaspoon onion powder
- 1/2 teaspoon black pepper
- 3 tablespoons crushed red pepper flakes
- 2 zucchinis, thinly sliced

Directions:

1. Mix oil with all the spices in a bowl.
2. Add zucchini slices and mix well.
3. Transfer the mixture to a Ziplock bag and seal it.
4. Refrigerate for 10 minutes.
5. Spread the zucchini slices on a greased baking sheet.
6. Bake for 15 minutes
7. Serve.

Nutrition:
Calories: 172
Fat: 11.1g
Carbs: 19.9g
Protein: 13.5g
Fiber: 0.2g

Apple Chips

Preparation Time: 5 minutes
Cooking Time: 45 minutes
Servings: 4
Ingredients:

- 2 Golden Delicious apples, cored and thinly sliced
- 1 1/2 teaspoons date sugar
- 1/2 teaspoon ground cinnamon

Directions:

1. Set your oven to 225 degrees F.
2. Place apple slices on a baking sheet.
3. Sprinkle sugar and cinnamon over apple slices.
4. Bake for 45 minutes.
5. Serve

Nutrition:

Calories: 127
Fat: 3.5g
Carbs: 33.6g
Protein: 4.5g
Fiber: 0.4g

Kale Crisps

Preparation Time: 10 minutes
Cooking Time: 10 minutes
Servings: 4
Ingredients:

- 1 bunch kale, stems removed, leaves torn into even pieces
- 1 tablespoon olive oil
- 1 teaspoon sea salt

Directions:

1. Set your oven to 350 degrees F. Layer a baking sheet with parchment paper.
2. Spread the kale leaves on a paper towel to absorb all the moisture.
3. Toss the leaves with sea salt, and olive oil.
4. Spread them on the baking sheet and bake for 10 minutes.
5. Serve.

Nutrition:

Calories: 113

Fat: 7.5g

Carbs: 1.4g

Protein: 1.1g

Fiber: 0g

Zucchini Chips

Preparation Time: 5 minutes

Cooking Time: 12 minutes

Servings: 4

Ingredients:

- 4 zucchinis, washed, peeled and sliced
- 2 teaspoons extra-virgin olive oil
- 1/4 teaspoon sea salt

Directions:

1. Set your oven to 350 degrees F.
2. Toss zucchinis with salt and olive oil.
3. Spread the slices on two baking sheets in a single layer.
4. Bake for 6 minutes on upper and lower rack of the oven.
5. Switch the baking racks and bake for another 6 minutes.
6. Serve.

Nutrition:

Calories: 153

Fat: 7.5g

Carbs: 20.4g

Protein: 3.1g

Fiber: 0g

Pita Chips

Preparation Time: 5 minutes
Cooking Time: 7 minutes
Servings: 4
Ingredients:

- 12 pita bread pockets, sliced into triangles
- 1/2 cup olive oil
- 1/2 teaspoon ground black pepper
- 1 teaspoon salt
- 1/2 teaspoon dried basil
- 1 teaspoon dried chervil

Directions:

1. Set your oven to 400 degrees F.
2. Toss pita with all the remaining ingredients in a bowl.
3. Spread the seasoned triangles on a baking sheet.
4. Bake for 7 minutes until golden brown.
5. Serve with your favorite hummus.

Nutrition:

Calories: 201
Fat: 5.5g
Carbs: 2.4g
Protein: 3.1g
Fiber: 0g

Turnip Chips

Preparation Time: 5 minutes
Cooking Time: 5 mins
Servings: 4
Ingredients:

- 1 turnip, thinly sliced
- 2 teaspoons olive oil, or as needed
- Coarse sea salt, to taste

Directions:

1. Toss turnip with oil and salt.
2. Spread the slices in a baking dish in a single layer.
3. Cook in a microwave for 5 minutes until golden brown.
4. Serve.

Nutrition:

Calories: 213

Fat: 8.5g

Carbs: 21.4g

Protein: 0.1g

Fiber: 0g

Chapter 22: Main Dishes

Kamut Burgers

Preparation Time: 20 minutes

Cooking Time: 20 minutes

Servings: 6

Ingredients:

- 3 cups cooked kamut cereal
- 1 cup spelt flour
- ½ cup unsweetened hemp milk
- 1 cup green bell peppers, seeded and chopped
- 1 cup red onions, chopped
- 1 tablespoon fresh oregano, chopped
- 1 tablespoon fresh basil, chopped
- 1 teaspoon onion powder
- 1 teaspoon sea salt
- ½ teaspoon cayenne powder
- 4 tablespoons grapeseed oil
- 8 cups fresh baby kale

Directions:

1. In a bowl, add all the ingredients except for oil and kale and mix until well combined.
2. Make 12 equal-sized patties from the mixture.
3. In a large skillet, heat 2 tablespoons of the oil over medium-high heat and cook 6 patties for about 4-5 minutes per side. Repeat with the remaining oil and patties.
4. Divide the kale onto serving plates and top each with 2 burgers.
5. Serve immediately.

Nutrition:
Calories: 459
Fat: 12.5g
Carbs: 80.6g
Protein: 16.4g
Fiber: 12.9g

Chickpeas & Mushroom Burgers
Preparation Time: 20 minutes
Cooking Time: 20 minutes
Servings: 4
Ingredients:

- 2 Portobello mushrooms, chopped roughly
- ½ cup green bell peppers, seeded and chopped roughly
- ½ cup white onion, chopped roughly
- 2 cups cooked chickpeas
- ½ cup fresh cilantro
- 2 teaspoons fresh oregano, chopped
- 2 teaspoons onion
- ½ teaspoon cayenne powder
- Sea salt, as required
- ¼ cup chickpea flour
- 3 tablespoons grapeseed oil

- 6 cups fresh baby arugula

Directions:

1. In a food processor place all of the ingredients and pulse for about 3 seconds.
2. Make 8 equal-sized patties from the mixture.
3. In a large skillet, heat half of the oil over medium-high heat and cook 4 patties for about 4-5 minutes per side.
4. Repeat with the remaining oil and patties.
5. Divide the arugula onto serving plates and top each with 2 burgers.
6. Serve immediately.

Nutrition:
Calories: 278
Fat: 12.2g
Carbs: 31g
Protein: 11.2g
Fiber: 7.6g

Veggie Burgers

Preparation Time: 0 minutes
Cooking Time: 6 minutes
Servings: 2
Ingredients:

- ½ cup fresh kale, tough ribs removed and chopped
- ½ cup green bell peppers, seeded and chopped
- ½ cup onions, chopped
- 1 plum tomato, chopped
- 2 teaspoons fresh oregano, chopped
- 2 teaspoons fresh basil, chopped
- 1 teaspoon dried dill

- 1 teaspoon onion powder
- ½ teaspoon ginger powder
- ½ teaspoon cayenne powder
- Sea salt, as required
- 1 cup chickpeas flour
- ¼–½ cup spring water
- 2 tablespoons grapeseed oil
- 3 cups fresh arugula

Directions:

1. In a large bowl, add the vegetables, herbs, spices, and salt and mix well.
2. Add the flour and mix well.
3. Slowly, add the water and mix until a thick mixture is formed.
4. Make desired-sized patties from the mixture.
5. In a large skillet, heat the oil over medium-high heat and cook the patties for about 2-3 minutes per side.
6. Divide the arugula onto serving plates and top each with 2 burgers.
7. Serve immediately.

Nutrition:
Calories: 354
Fat: 17.8g
Carbs: 38.4g
Protein: 13g
Fiber: 8.1g

Falafel with Tzatziki Sauce
Preparation Time: 20 minutes
Cooking Time: 12 minutes
Servings: 8
Ingredients:

For Falafel

- 1 pound dry chickpeas, soaked overnight, drained, and rinsed
- 1 small onion, chopped roughly
- ¼ cup fresh parsley, chopped
- 4 garlic cloves, peeled
- 1½ tablespoons chickpea flour
- Sea salt, as required
- ½ teaspoon cayenne powder
- ½ cup grapeseed oil

For Tzatziki Sauce

- ½ cup Brazil nuts, soaked in spring water for 6-8 hours
- ½ cup spring water
- ¼ cup cucumber, chopped
- 1 tablespoon fresh key lime juice
- 1 garlic clove, minced
- 1 teaspoon fresh dill
- Pinch of sea salt

For Serving

- 12 cups fresh arugula

Directions:
For Falafel

1. In a food processor, add all the ingredients and pulse until well combined and coarse meal like mixture forms.
2. Transfer the falafel mixture into a bowl.
3. With a plastic wrap, cover the bowl and refrigerate for about 1-2 hours.
4. With 2 tablespoons of the mixture, make balls.

5. In a large skillet, heat the oil to 375 degrees F.
6. Add the falafels in 2 batches and cook for about 5-6 minutes or until golden brown from all aides.
7. Meanwhile, for tzatziki: in a blender, add all the ingredients and pulse until smooth.
8. With a slotted spoon, transfer the falafels onto a paper towel-lined plate to drain.
9. Divide the arugula and falafels onto serving plates evenly.
10. Serve alongside the tzatziki.

Nutrition:
Calories: 283
Fat: 9.6g
Carbs: 38.8g
Protein: 13.3g
Fiber: 11.3g

Veggie Balls in Tomato Sauce
Preparation Time: 20 minutes
Cooking Time: 15 minutes
Servings: 8
Ingredients:

- 1½ cups cooked chickpeas
- 2 cups fresh button mushrooms
- ½ cup onions, chopped
- ¼ cup green bell peppers, seeded and chopped
- 2 teaspoons oregano
- 2 teaspoons fresh basil
- 1 teaspoon savory
- 1 teaspoon dried sage

- 1 teaspoon dried dill
- 1 tablespoon onion powder
- ½ teaspoon cayenne powder
- ½ teaspoon ginger powder
- Sea salt, as required
- ½-1 cup chickpea flour
- 6 cups homemade tomato sauce
- 2 tablespoons grapeseed oil

Directions:

1. In a food processor, add the chickpeas, veggies, herbs and spices and pulse until well combined.
2. Transfer the mixture into a large bowl with flour and mix until well combined.
3. Make desired-sized balls from the mixture.
4. In a large skillet, heat the oil over medium-high heat and cook the balls in 2 batches for about 4-5 minutes or until golden brown from all sides.
5. In a large pan, add the tomato sauce and veggie balls over medium heat and simmer for about 5 minutes.
6. Serve hot.

Nutrition:
Calories: 159
Fat: 4.8g
Carbs: 23.9g
Protein: 7.2g
Fiber: 6g

Veggie Kabobs
Preparation Time: 20 minutes
Cooking Time: 10 minutes

Servings: 4
Ingredients:
For Marinade

- 2 garlic cloves, minced
- 2 teaspoons fresh basil, minced
- 2 teaspoons fresh oregano, minced
- ½ teaspoon cayenne powder
- Sea salt, as required
- 2 tablespoons fresh key lime juice
- 2 tablespoons avocado oil

For Veggies

- 2 large zucchinis, cut into thick slices
- 8 large button mushrooms, quartered
- 1 yellow bell pepper, seeded and cubed
- 1 red bell pepper, seeded and cubed

Directions:

1. For marinade: in a large bowl, add all the ingredients and mix until well combined. Add the vegetables and toss to coat well.
2. Cover and refrigerate to marinate for at least 6-8 hours. Preheat the grill to medium-high heat. Generously, grease the grill grate.
3. Remove the vegetables from the bowl and thread onto pre-soaked wooden skewers.
4. Grill for about 8-10 minutes or until done completely, flipping occasionally.

Nutrition:

Calories: 122

Fat: 7.8g

Carbs: 12.7g

Protein: 4.3g

Fiber: 3.5g

Spiced Okra

Preparation time: 10 minutes

Cooking time: 13 minutes

Servings: 2

Ingredients:

- 1 tablespoon avocado oil
- ¾ pound okra pods, trimmed and cut into 2-inch pieces
- ½ teaspoon ground cumin
- ½ teaspoon cayenne powder
- Sea salt, as required

Directions:

1. In a large skillet, heat the oil over medium heat and stir fry the okra and stir fry for about 2 minutes.
2. Reduce the heat to low and cook covered for about 6-8 minutes stirring occasionally.
3. Add the cumin, cayenne powder and salt and stir to combine.
4. Increase the heat to medium and cook uncovered for about 2-3 minutes more.
5. Remove from the heat and serve hot.

Nutrition:

Calories: 81

Fat: 1.4g

Carbs: 13.5g

Protein: 3.5g

Fiber: 5.9g

Mushroom Curry

Preparation Time: 15 minutes

Cooking Time: 25 minutes

Servings: 4

Ingredients:

- 2 cups plum tomatoes, chopped
- 2 tablespoons grapeseed oil
- 1 small onion, chopped finely
- ¼ teaspoon cayenne powder
- 4 cups fresh button mushrooms, sliced
- 1¼ cups spring water
- ¼ cup unsweetened coconut milk
- Sea salt, as required

Directions:

1. In a food processor, add the tomatoes and pulse until a smooth paste forms.
2. In a pan, heat the oil over medium heat and sauté the onion for about 5-6 minutes.
3. Add the tomato paste and cook for about 5 minutes. Stir in the mushrooms, water and coconut milk and bring to a boil.
4. Cook for about 10-12 minutes, stirring occasionally. Season with the salt and remove from the heat.
5. Serve hot.

Nutrition:

Calories: 126
Fat: 9.5g
Carbs: 9g
Protein: 3.7g
Fiber: 2.1g

Bell Peppers & Zucchini Stir Fry

Preparation time: 15 minutes
Cooking time: 15 minutes
Servings: 4
Ingredients:

- 2 tablespoons avocado oil
- 1 large onion, cubed
- 4 garlic cloves, minced
- 1 large green bell pepper, seeded and cubed
- 1 large red bell pepper, seeded and cubed
- 1 large yellow bell pepper, seeded and cubed
- 2 cups zucchini, sliced
- ¼ cup spring water
- Sea salt, as required
- Cayenne powder, as required

Directions:

1. In a large skillet, heat the oil over medium heat and sauté the onion and garlic for about 4-5 minutes.
2. Add the vegetables and stir fry for about 4-5 minutes.
3. Add the water and stir fry for about 3-4 minutes more.
4. Serve hot.

Nutrition:

Calories: 66

Fat: 1.3g

Carbs: 13.5g

Protein: 2.3g

Fiber: 3g;

Yellow Squash & Bell Pepper Bake

Preparation Time: 15 minutes

Cooking Time: 20 minutes

Servings: 4

Ingredients:

- 2 large yellow squash, chopped
- 1 large red bell pepper, seeded and cubed
- 1 large yellow bell peppers, seeded and cubed
- 1 onion, cubed
- 1 tablespoon agave nectar
- 2 tablespoons grapeseed oil
- 1 teaspoon cayenne powder
- Sea salt, as required

Directions:

1. Preheat the oven to 375 degrees F. Lightly, grease a large baking dish.
2. In a large bowl, add all the ingredients and mix well.
3. Transfer the vegetable mixture into the prepared baking dish.
4. Bake for about 15-20 minutes.
5. Remove from the oven and serve immediately.

Nutrition:

Calories: 132

Fat: 7.6g

Carbs: 16.7g

Protein: 2.9g

Fiber: 3.5g

Mushrooms with Bell Peppers

Preparation time: 15 minutes

Cooking time: 10 minutes

Servings: 2

Ingredients:

- 1 tablespoon grapeseed oil
- 3 cups fresh button mushrooms, sliced
- ¾ cups red bell peppers, seeded and cut into long strips
- ¾ cups green bell peppers, seeded and cut into long strips
- 1½ cup white onions, cut into long strips
- 2 teaspoons fresh sweet basil
- 2 teaspoons fresh oregano
- ½ teaspoon cayenne powder
- Sea salt, as required
- 2 teaspoons onion powder

Directions:

1. In a large skillet, heat the oil over medium-high heat and sauté the mushrooms, bell peppers, and onion for about 5-6 minutes.
2. Add the herbs and spices and cook for about 2-3 minutes. Stir in the lime juice and serve hot.

Nutrition:

Calories: 80

Fat: 3.9g

Carbs: 10.7g

Protein: 2.8g
Fiber: 2.5g

24

Chapter 23: Soup Recipes

Turnip Green Soup

Preparation Time: 5 minutes.

Cooking Time: 22 minutes.

Servings: 2

Ingredients:

- 2 tbsps. Coconut oil
- 1 large chopped onion
- 3 minced cloves chive
- 2—in piece peeled and minced ginger
- 3 cups bone broth
- 1 medium cubed white turnip
- 1 large chopped head radish
- 1 bunch chopped kale
- 1 Seville orange, 1/2 zested and juice reserved
- 1/2 tsp. sea salt
- 1 bunch cilantro

Directions:

1. In a skillet, add oil then heat it.
2. Add in the onions as you stir.
3. Sauté for about 7 minutes, then add chive and ginger.
4. Cook for about 1 minute.
5. Add in the turnip, broth, and radish then stir.
6. Bring the soup to boil then reduce the heat to allow it to simmer.
7. Cook for an extra 15 minutes then turn off the heat.
8. Pour in the remaining ingredients.
9. Using a handheld blender, pour the mixture.
10. Garnish with cilantro.
11. Serve warm.

Nutrition:

Calories: 249 kcal.

Fat: 11.9g.

Carbs: 1.8g.

Protein: 35g

Fiber: 0g

Lentil Kale Soup

Preparation Time: 5 minutes

Cooking Time: 15 minutes.

Servings: 4

Ingredients:

- 1/2 Onion
- 2 Zucchinis
- 1 rib Celery
- 1 stalk Chive
- 1 cup diced tomatoes
- 1 tsp. dried vegetable broth powder
- 1 tsp. Sazon seasoning
- 1 cup red lentils

- 1 tbsp. Seville orange juice
- 3 cups alkaline water
- 1 bunch kale

Directions:

1. In a greased pan, pour in all the vegetables.
2. Sauté for about 5 minutes, then add the tomatoes, broth, and Sazon seasoning.
3. Mix properly then stir in the red lentils together with water.
4. Cook until the lentils become soft and tender.
5. Add the kale then cook for about 2 minutes.
6. Serve warm with the Seville orange juice.

Nutrition:
Calories: 301
Fat: 12.2g
Carbs: 15g
Protein: 28.8g
Fiber: 0g

Tangy Lentil Soup
Preparation time: 5 minutes
Cooking time: 15 minutes
Servings: 4
Ingredients:

- 2 cups picked over and rinsed red lentils
- 1 chopped serrano Chile pepper
- 1 large chopped and roughly tomato
- 1-1/2 inch peeled and grated piece ginger
- 3 finely chopped cloves chive

- 1/4 tsp. ground turmeric
- Sea salt

Topping

- 1/4 cup coconut yogurt

Directions:

1. In a pot add the lentils with enough water to cover the lentils.
2. Boil the lentils then reduce the heat.
3. Cook for about 10 minutes on low heat to simmer.
4. Add the remaining ingredients then stir.
5. Cook until lentils become soft and properly mixed.
6. Garnish a dollop of coconut yogurt.
7. Serve.

Nutrition:

Calories: 248 kcal.
Fat: 2.4g.
Carbs: 12.2g.
Protein: 44.3g.
Fiber: 0g

Vegetable Casserole

Preparation Time: 5 minutes.
Cooking Time: 1 hour 30 minutes.
Servings: 6
Ingredients:

- 2 large peeled and sliced eggplants
- Sea salt

- 2 large diced cucumbers
- 2 small diced green peppers
- 1 Small diced red pepper
- 1 Small diced yellow pepper
- 1/4 lb. sliced green beans
- 1/2 cup olive oil
- 2 large chopped sweet onions
- 3 crushed cloves chive
- 2 cubed yellow Squash,
- 20 halved cherry tomatoes
- 1/2 tsp. sea salt
- 1/4 tsp. fresh ground pepper
- 1/4 cup alkaline water
- 1 cup fresh seasoned breadcrumbs

Directions:

1. Adjust the temperature of your oven to 350°F.
2. Mix the eggplant with salt then keep it aside.
3. Heat a greased skillet then sautés the eggplant until it is evenly browned.
4. Transfer the eggplant to a separate plate.
5. Sauté the onions in the same pan until it becomes soft.
6. Add the chive then stir.
7. Cook for a minute then turn off the heat.
8. Layer a greased casserole dish with the eggplants, yellow squash, cucumbers, peppers, and green beans.
9. Add the onion mixture, tomatoes, pepper, and salt.
10. Sprinkle the seasoned breadcrumbs as toppings.
11. Bake for an hour and 30 minutes.
12. Serve.

Nutrition:

Calories: 372 kcal

Fat: 11.1g

Carbs: 0.9g

Protein: 63.5g

Fiber: 0g

Mushroom Leek Soup

Preparation time: 5 minutes.

Cooking Time: 8 minutes.

Servings: 4

Ingredients:

- 3 tbsps. Divided vegetable oil
- 2—3/4 cups finely chopped leeks
- 3 finely minced chive stalks
- 7 cups cleaned and sliced assorted mushrooms
- 5 tbsps. Coconut flour
- 3/4 tsp. sea salt
- 1/2 tsp. ground black pepper
- 1 tbsp. finely minced fresh dill
- 3 cups vegetable broth
- 2/3 cup coconut cream
- 1/2 cup coconut milk
- 1—1/2 tbsps. Sherry vinegar

Directions:

1. Preheat oil in a Dutch oven, then sauté the leeks and chive until they become soft.
2. Add in the mushrooms then stir.
3. Sauté for about 10 minutes.
4. Add pepper, dill, flour, and salt.
5. Mix properly then cook for about 2 minutes.

6. Pour in the broth then cook to boil.
7. Reduce the heat in the oven then add the remaining ingredients.
8. Serve warm with coconut flour bread.

Nutrition:

Calories: 127 kcal.

Fat: 3.5g.

Carbs: 3.6g.

Protein: 21.5g.

Fiber: 0g

Red Lentil Squash Soup

Preparation Time: 5 minutes

Cooking Time: 4 minutes

Servings: 4

Ingredients:

- 1 chopped yellow onion
- 2 tbsps. Olive oil
- 1 large diced butternut squash
- 1—1/2 cups red lentils
- 2 tsps. Dried sage
- 7 cups vegetable broth
- Mineral sea salt & white or fresh cracked pepper

Directions:

1. Preheat the oil in a stockpot.
2. Add the onions then cook for about 5 minutes.
3. Add in the sage and squash.
4. Cook for 5 minutes.
5. Add broth, pepper, lentils, and salt.

6. Cook gradually for 30 minutes on low heat.
7. Pour the mixture using a handheld blender.
8. Garnish with cilantro.
9. Serve.

Nutrition:

Calories: 323 kcal.

Fat: 7.5g.

Carbs: 21.4g.

Protein: 10.1g

Fiber: 0g

Cauliflower Potato Curry

Preparation Time: 10 minutes.

Cooking Time: 35 minutes.

Servings: 4

Ingredients:

- 2 tbsps. Vegetable oil
- 1 large chopped onion
- A large grated piece of ginger
- 3 finely chopped chive stalks
- 1/2 tsp. turmeric
- 1 tsp. ground cumin
- 1 tsp. curry powder
- 1 cup chopped tomatoes
- 1/2 tsp. sugar
- 1 florets cauliflower
- 2 chopped potatoes
- 1 small halved lengthways green chili
- A squeeze Seville orange juice
- Handful roughly chopped coriander

Directions:

1. Add the onion to a greased skillet then sauté until soft.
2. Add all the spices in the skillet then stir.
3. Add the cauliflower and potatoes.
4. Sauté for about 5 minutes, then add green chilies tomatoes, and sugar.
5. Cover then cook for about 30 minutes.
6. Serve warm with the coriander and Seville orange juice.

Nutrition:

Calories: 332 kcal.
Fat: 7.5g.
Carbs: 19.4g.
Protein: 3.1g
Fiber: 0g

Vegetable Bean Curry

Preparation Time: 5 minutes
Cooking Time: 6 hours
Servings: 8
Ingredients:

- 1 finely chopped onion
- 4 chopped chive stalks
- 3 tsps. Coriander powder
- 1/2 tsp. cinnamon powder
- 1 tsp. ginger powder
- 1 tsp. turmeric powder
- 1/2 tsp. cayenne pepper
- 2 tbsps. Tomato paste
- 1 tbsp. avocado oil
- 2 cans, 15 ounces each, well rinsed and drained lima beans

- 3 cups cubed and peeled turnips
- 3 cups fresh cauliflower florets
- 4 medium diced zucchinis
- 2 medium seeded and chopped tomatoes
- 2 cups vegetable broth
- 1 cup light coconut milk
- 1/2 tsp. pepper
- 1/4 tsp. sea salt

Directions:

1. In a slow cooker, preheat the oil then add all the vegetables.
2. Add in the remaining ingredients then stir.
3. Cook for about 6 hours on low-temperature.
4. Serve warm.

Nutrition:

Calories: 403 kcal

Fat: 12.5g

Carbs: 21.4g

Protein: 8.1g

Fiber: 0g

Wild Mushroom Soup

Preparation Time: 10 minutes

Cooking Time: 15 minute

Servings: 4

Ingredients:

- 4 oz. walnut butter
- 1 chopped shallot
- 5 oz. chopped portabella mushrooms

- 5 oz. chopped oyster mushrooms
- 5 oz. chopped shiitake mushrooms
- 1 minced chive clove
- 1/2 tsp. dried thyme
- 3 cups alkaline water
- 1 vegetable bouillon cube
- 1 cup coconut cream
- 1/2 lb. chopped celery root
- 1 tbsp. white wine vinegar
- Fresh cilantro

Directions:

1. In a cooking pan, melt the butter over medium heat.
2. Add the vegetables into the pan then sauté until golden brown.
3. Add the remaining ingredients to the pan then properly mix it.
4. Boil the mixture.
5. Simmer it for 15 minutes on low heat.
6. Add the cream to the soup then pour it using a hand-held blender.
7. Serve warm with the chopped cilantro as toppings.

Nutrition:

Calories: 243 kcal

Fat: 7.5g

Carbs: 14.4g

Protein: 10.1g

Fiber: 0g

Bok Choy Soup

Preparation Time: 5 minutes.

Cooking Time: 10 minutes.

Servings: 2

Ingredients:

- 1 cup chopped Bok Choy
- 3 cups vegetable broth
- 2 peeled and sliced zucchinis
- 1/2 cup cooked hemp seed
- 1 roughly chopped bunch radish

Directions:

1. In a pan, mix the ingredients over moderate heat.
2. Let it simmer then cook it for about 10 minutes until the vegetables become tender.
3. Serve.

Nutrition:

Calories: 172 kcal.
Fat: 3.5g
Carbs: 38.5g
Protein: 11.7g
Fiber: 0g

Grilled Vegetable Stack

Preparation Time: 10 minutes
Cooking Time: 20 minutes
Servings: 2
Ingredients:

- 1/2 zucchini, sliced into slices about 1/4—inch thick
- 2 stemmed Portobello mushrooms with the gills removed
- 1 tsp. divided sea salt
- 1/2 cup divided hummus
- 1 peeled and sliced red onion

- 1 seeded red bell pepper, sliced lengthwise
- 1 seeded yellow bell pepper, sliced lengthwise

Directions:

1. Adjust the temperature of your broiler or grill.
2. Grill the mushroom caps over coal or gas flame.
3. Add the yellow and red bell peppers, onion, and zucchini for about 20 minutes as you turn it occasionally.
4. Fill the mushroom cap with 1/4 cup of hummus.
5. Top it with some onion, yellow peppers, red and zucchini.
6. Add salt to season then set it aside.
7. Redo the process with the second mushroom cap and the remaining ingredients.
8. Serve.

Nutrition:

Calories: 179 kcal

Fat: 3.1g

Carbs: 15.7g

Protein: 3.9g

Fiber: 0g

Date Night Chive Bake

Preparation Time: 10 minutes.

Cooking Time: 30 minutes.

Servings: 2

Ingredients:

- 4 peeled and sliced lengthwise zucchinis
- 1 lb. Radish chopped into bite-size pieces
- 2 tsps. Seville orange zest

- 3 peeled and chopped chive heads cloves
- 2 tbsps. Coconut oil
- 1 cup vegetable broth
- 1/4 tsps. Mustard powder
- 1 tsp. sea salt

Directions:

1. Adjust the temperature of the oven to 400°F. In a separate bowl, mix all the ingredients.
2. Spread the mixture in a baking pan evenly. Cover the mixture with a piece of aluminum foil then place it in the oven.
3. Bake the mixture for about 30 minutes as you stir it once halfway through the cooking time.

Nutrition:
Calories: 270 kcal
Fat: 15.2g
Carbs: 28.1g
Protein: 11.6g
Fiber: 0g

Champions Chili
Preparation Time: 5 minutes
Cooking Time: 25 minutes
Servings: 4
Ingredients:

- 1 cup diced red bell pepper
- 1 chopped onion
- 2 finely chopped chive stalks
- 2 cups sprouted pinto beans

- 1/4 cup fresh organic cilantro
- 1/4 cup organic salsa
- 8 oz. jar organic pasta sauce
- 2 tbsps. Barbecue sauce
- Dash of ground cumin
- Dash of chili powder

Directions:

1. Apply some non-stick cooking spray to a pot.
2. Place the pot over a moderate heat then sauté the onion for about 5 minutes.
3. Add in the ingredients then stir. Simmer for about 20 minutes.
4. Serve.

Nutrition:

Calories: 101 kcal

Fat: 2.7g

Carbs: 18.5g

Protein: 3.9g

Fiber: 0g

25

Conclusion

The alkaline diet is very healthy and encourages participants to eat more vegetables and healthy plant foods while restricting how they consume processed junk foods. These plants and herbs are nature's gift to man for treating several diseases and illnesses at a lesser cost than pharmaceutical drugs. In my book, Herbal Medicines, I discussed intensively the medicinal herbs we have, their uses, and how they can be applied to achieve a maximum result.

The Alkaline diet is considered safe because it is all about consuming whole and unprocessed foods.

However, the healthiest diet option is one that is rich in variety. It is important to go for a diet that has a range of different grains, proteins, vitamins, vegetables, fruits, and minerals.

When you remove any single food type or group from a diet, it may make it difficult to be healthy. Although a very low protein alkaline diet can help you lose weight, it may also increase the risk of having other weak muscles and bones. Ensure to get enough protein while on the alkaline diet. Once you are sure of getting enough protein from the alkaline diet, you can begin this diet.

Dr. Sebi's alkaline diet is a popular diet made for curing illnesses that have been followed by many people. But scientific studies do not show that it results in curing any type of chronic disease. It is now seen as a method to lose weight and follow a healthy lifestyle to improve overall health.

Dr. Sebi's was a self-proclaimed herbalist who coined this diet. He has a questionable background and education when it comes to healing people. The diet is very restrictive and difficult to follow, even more, difficult than vegan dieting.

It can provide all the benefits that a low-calorie and high fresh vegetable and fruit diet can give. The benefits are enormous, but the level of calories should wander close to the calories you burn on average, or else you will feel lethargic, and a process called cell starvation will start. However, if your main goal is to reduce weight, it can give promising results.

Trying different diets is a way to find out what type suits you. If you need fast weight loss and don't mind the restrictions, then this diet can be for you. To achieve the goals that you desire, you need to sacrifice some comforts of your life. We are used to being in bad routines because they don't require any effort. If we want to live healthily, we need to put some sort of effort and hard work into it.

The list of approved foods may not look like a lot to you, but it contains a variety of ingredients that can lead to great meals. However, if you think that you cannot handle this diet, start the diet slowly by replacing one meal a week and then gradually improving.

Good luck to everyone who has decided to embark on the journey of alkaline dieting! I hope that you carefully follow the instructions of this diet to get closer to your desires and healthy life!

Made in the USA
Las Vegas, NV
07 January 2025

16012557R00098